SUGAR**DETOX**ME

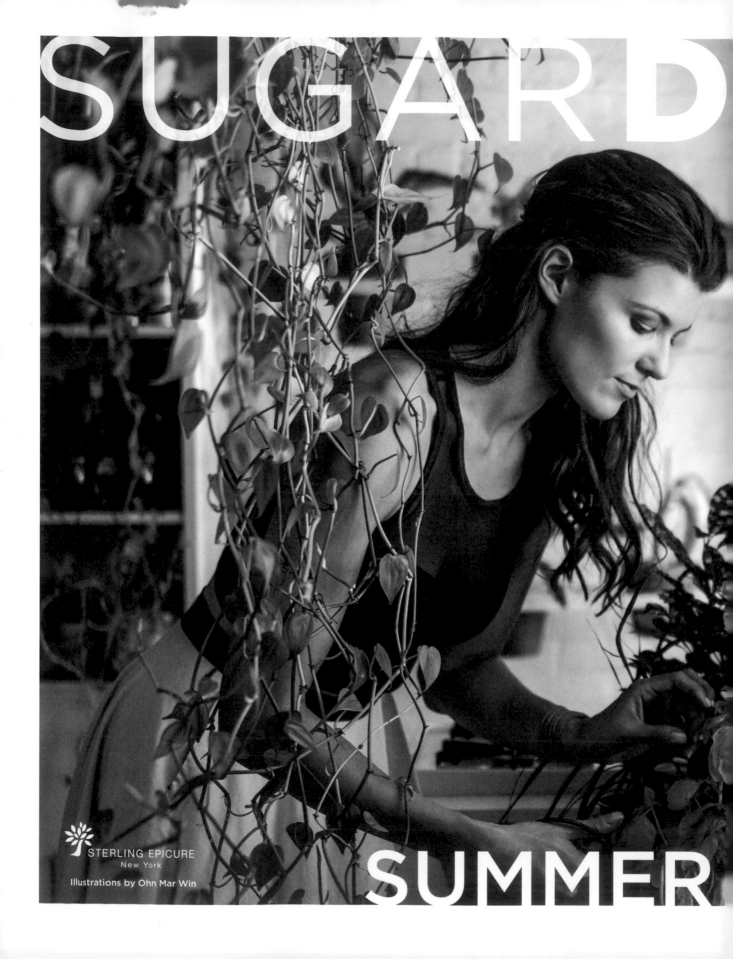

SUGAR

SUMMER

STERLING EPICURE
New York

Illustrations by Ohn Mar Win

ETOXME

100+ Recipes
to Curb Cravings
& Take Back
Your Health

RAYNE OAKES

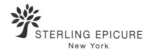

STERLING EPICURE
New York

An Imprint of Sterling Publishing Co., Inc.
1166 Avenue of the Americas
New York, NY 10036

Library of Congress Cataloging-in-Publication Data

Names: Oakes, Summer Rayne, author.
Title: Sugardetoxme : 100+ recipes to curb cravings and take back your health / Summer Rayne Oakes.
Description: New York City : Sterling Epicure, [2017]
Identifiers: LCCN 2016051540 | ISBN 9781454923053 (hardback)
Subjects: LCSH: Sugar-free diet--Popular works. | Detoxification
  (Health)--Popular works. | Weight loss--Popular works. | BISAC: COOKING /
  Health & Healing / General.
Classification: LCC RM237.85 .O25 2017 | DDC 641.5/63837--dc23
LC record available at https://lccn.loc.gov/2016051540

ISBN 978-1-4549-2305-3

Distributed in Canada by Sterling Publishing Co., Inc.
c/o Canadian Manda Group, 664 Annette Street
Toronto, Ontario, Canada M6S 2C8
Distributed in the United Kingdom by GMC Distribution Services
Castle Place, 166 High Street, Lewes, East Sussex, England BN7 1XU
Distributed in Australia by NewSouth Books
45 Beach Street, Coogee, NSW 2034, Australia

For information about custom editions, special sales, and premium and corporate purchases,
please contact Sterling Special Sales at 800-805-5489 or specialsales@sterlingpublishing.com.

Manufactured in Canada

2 4 6 8 10 9 7 5 3 1

www.sterlingpublishing.com

Design by Lorie Pagnozzi
Photography on pages ii-iii, xii, xviii-1, 35, 54-55, 238 by Joey L.
Recipe icons and charts on page 242: Shutterstock

INTRODUCTION

About three years ago, while working on sustainable food systems, I began a journey to understand why I craved sugar so much. This curiosity and the need to know how to overcome my seemingly innate sugar habit led me on a Nancy Drew–like investigation. I began researching all I could about our relationship to the sweet stuff and how it got into our food system in the first place.

When I first did a sugar cleanse, I did it just for me. I felt like my sugar tooth was the one thing that was standing in my way to become optimally healthy, and I wanted to get a handle on it. I decided to design a guide that I could stick to, that would keep me honest, and that I could turn to again and again, if I ever fell off track, until it became a way of life. In short, the focus on sugar in my own diet was a lens that helped clarify and define my vision of a healthier life—one that I'd like to pass along to you.

I started documenting my sugar cleanse via my website SugarDetox.me, which later led to an easy-to-follow, empowering program to help others do the same. When I set out on my journey, I didn't expect that so many people would be interested in doing it with me. Some of their reasons were different from mine, because eating too much sugar can have varied and far-reaching health effects, everything from energy dips to skin problems to cavities to metabolic disorders such as diabetes, nonalcoholic fatty liver disease, and even gout.

Let's backtrack, though. Even though I considered myself a healthy eater in general, it wouldn't be uncommon for me to eat half a box of cookies in one sitting, if they were just lying around. Luckily, I rarely purchased sweets at the store or made them at home, but when I did, they wouldn't last long! Sound familiar?

I really wanted to get to the root cause of what was driving me to eat sugar in such quantities. Most of the sugary stuff that I was eating had zero nutritional value, too. I repeat: *zero*, which means I wasn't getting any health benefits whatsoever or any vital amino acids, vitamins, or minerals to fuel my brain and body. It was a total drag for someone who considers herself healthy, relatively speaking. Plus, I was the kid of two health-conscious parents, but unlike my mom and dad (or my brother for that matter), I was the one saddled with the sweet tooth.

I ATE THE CHRISTMAS LIGHTS

Even before I was able to comprehend the consequences of certain eating habits, I was drawn like a magnet to sweet-looking foods. One Christmas, to my mother's horror, two-year-old me reached into a green glass bowl of colored Christmas lights that I could barely get to on my tiptoes. Thinking they were a friendly relative of Skittles® or some other Willy Wonka–esque candy, I began to crunch the glass bulbs. My mother screamed, which immediately halted my treacherous actions. "Open your mouth," she commanded. "Don't swallow anything." And then she quickly ushered me to the emergency room, without any major damage.

Even when I was aware of the consequences, however, I struggled to curb my almost inexorable desire for sweets. Even as I'm writing this, it's unbelievable how vivid the memories are around my obsession with sweet stuff. At my cousin's birthday party as a five-year-old, I recall that I knowingly

"stole" his bag of candy and proceeded to eat everything, from powdered candy in a straw to gummy worms. As I reminisce, I can even remember what I was wearing; I can see my mother scolding me in the gravel driveway, and taste the tartness of the powder on my tongue. The theft of the candy resulted in tears from my cousin and for me, a reprimand from my mother.

Years later, there was an even more embarrassing event, which involved caching sweets from the candy bowl at my piano teacher's house. I would arrive early for my lesson, remove my shoes, and give my teacher her check. She would then take the check to another room and wouldn't come back to the piano until it was officially time for the lesson to start. I made it a point to have my mother drop me off early so that gave me more time to raid the big candy bowl in my teacher's living room. If I didn't have pockets, I would stuff the candies beneath the seat cushions of her couch so that I could covertly remove them while putting on my shoes before heading home.

I was, of course, a little embarrassed to take any candy from the bowl while she was in the living room, because, after all, I couldn't take just one. Hence the stash technique. Like a fugitive, I would hide the candy under the cushion and without fail walk away with handfuls of the sweet contraband.

I would have probably forgotten about this recurring episode except that one day the routine changed. My piano teacher's mother, knowing our lesson wasn't going to start for another ten minutes, decided to vacuum the living room. I fretted. Just two minutes before, I'd stuffed a heaping handful of hard candy into the corner of the couch. What if she picked up the couch cushion—like my mother did at home—to clean up any crumbs?

I tried to act calm, but I was getting nervous and

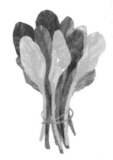

To all those who are willing to trade in their sweet tooth in exchange for a healthier life. And to my family and friends—with whom I've shared many delicious meals and engaging conversations about life, love, and living.

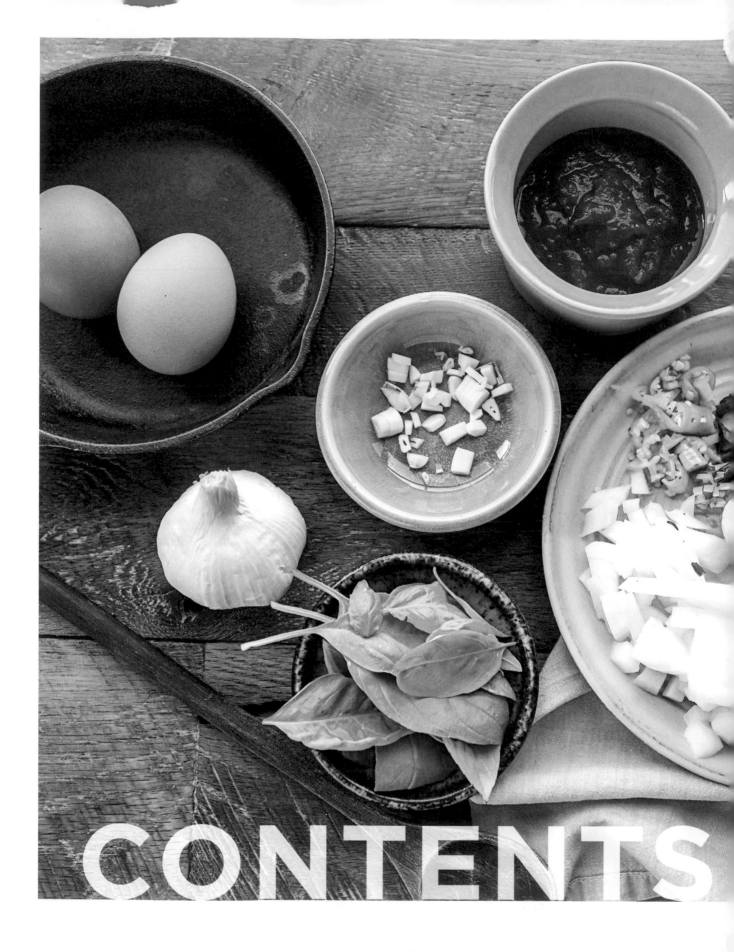

CONTENTS

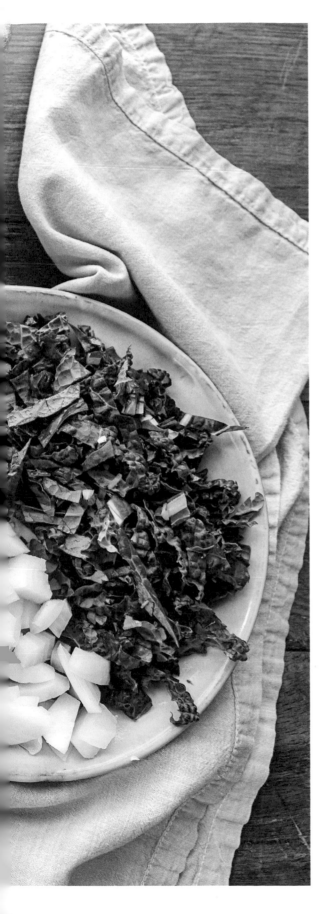

FOREWORD

Whatever has brought you to this book, congratulations! In its pages you will get the inspiration you need to embrace a new relationship with sugar. Whether you're like Summer Rayne—and were born with a sweet tooth, one you've been nursing for a long time—or simply someone who is curious about how to reduce your intake of sugar in an environment where the stuff is ubiquitous, this book is an invaluable resource.

My own sugar epiphany happened fifteen years ago. Despite having been raised by a mom who is considered the godmother of healthy eating—the woman who penned the vegetarian bible, *Diet for a Small Planet*—I myself had become far from a paragon of healthy eating. I was living on the Upper West Side of Manhattan, surviving graduate school on a shoestring budget. I tried, but more often than not, failed, to eat well, especially when it came to what I drank.

I was spending many late nights in the library devouring econ textbooks and early mornings in classes scribbling notes, fueling it all with sugary drinks. Some days, I would have just one. But on many days I was drinking two, even three, in a day.

Back then I didn't know much about the sugary-drinks industry and its impact on people and the planet. I didn't realize the implications of the 20-ounce, hot pink, Power-C VitaminWater® I was drinking that contained 31 grams of sugar or the 16-ounce Organic Mango Nantucket Nectar® that contained 58 grams of sugar, according to the labels. I had no idea that with just one drink I was maxing out the sugar I should have been consuming in an entire day. (The American Heart Association recommends that women consume no more than 24 grams of added sugar a day). On the days when I would have a few drinks, I was easily consuming the equivalent of several *tablespoons* of sugar!

I also didn't know, then, what the effect of that liquid sugar was on my body—the effects of which you'll learn more about in these pages. I had yet to learn, for instance, that sugary drinks are the single largest source of added sugars in our diets and a leading cause of heart disease, liver disease, and type 2 diabetes. I had yet to understand how liquid sugar overwhelms our body's natural mechanisms for processing sugar and can lead to chronic diseases, from fatty liver disease to diabetes, or that consuming just one or two sugary drinks in a day can increase your chances of developing type 2 diabetes by 26 percent.

I didn't have Summer's book to guide me, but I did have a French boyfriend. Among the things that shocked him about this country were what we Americans drink. At our local bodega, the bursting beverage aisle flabbergasted Eric. "Why would you drink anything but water, espresso, and wine?" he asked me, genuinely perplexed.

Eric gave me a challenge that verged on an ultimatum: Drop the drinks. At first, I didn't think I could. I had been swayed by marketing, believing my bubbly personality and stamina were inextricably linked to those beverages. I would read my political science texts, highlighter pen in hand and a VitaminWater "Focus" on my desk (31 grams of sugar), and then power through accounting problems with an Odwalla Vanilla Protein Shake® an arm's reach away (43 grams of sugar).

But I took the leap. And, as you'll read in these pages, taking the leap is the first step to wean your-self off sugar. In my case, I was motivated not only by Eric, but by some simple math: I was easily spending $5 a day, or more, on drinks alone. As a struggling graduate student, every dollar counted. Not long after my cold turkey decision, I found that I was not only saving money, but also effortlessly shedding the pounds I'd put on as an undergrad—arriving at a set point I've kept, except for my two pregnancies, ever since. I felt better; I had *more* energy, not less. I've never looked back.

I rarely told the story of my sugar-kicking moment; when I did, I would do so with eyes cast down, embarrassed. I'm over that now: I think it's important that *no one* feel ashamed of where he or she falls along the sugar-consuming spectrum. We've got to be kind to ourselves. Remember, the food industry, particularly Big Soda, spends billions every year convincing us to want what they sell. Even the most strong-willed of us can't help but be influenced. That's why we need books like this one, and communities like the one Summer is building.

As you will learn through Summer's pep talks throughout this fabulous book, ditching sugar isn't necessarily as hard as you might think—and there are countless reasons why it's a good idea. We're learning more all the time about what sugar, and sugar-sweetened beverages, do to our bodies—the bodies of children, teens, and adults all around the world. We know that just one 12-ounce can of most sodas gives kids twice the grams of added sugar that the World Health Organization recommends they consume in an entire day. We know that diabetes is burdening our health care system in the United States with $245 billion in costs every year. And we know what the soda industry is doing to fight common sense policy measures, like sugary drinks taxes, a battle we actually won—in a landside—in my own small city of Berkeley, California.

We know of other reasons to turn our back on sugar: the environmental toll of sugar production, for instance. Worldwide sugar cane and sugar beet production—the two main sources of sugars in processed foods and sugary drinks—is a huge driver of biodiversity loss and water and air pollution. Sugar production in places like Florida have created massive environmental problems, like the pollution that is now choking the state's Lake Okeechobee, resulting in billions of dollars in cleanup costs.

But no matter what the motivation for kicking your sugar habit may be, this book will guide you.

It's a great time to rethink your relationship to sugar: You are not alone. All around the world, communities are waking up to the harmful impact of eating and drinking so much sugar. They're taking action, from campaigns to tax sugary drinks or put health-warning labels on soda, to launching education campaigns on the harms of sugar. And the great news is you don't have to wait until public policy catches up to common sense: You can take control of sugar in your own life, today, right now. This book is a great way to start.

Whether you go cold turkey or just cut sugary drinks out of your diet, you can do so knowing you are helping the environment and improving your health at the same time. Summer's book gives you the inspiration and practical tips to embrace health and kick out Big Sugar—your body and the planet will thank you.

—ANNA LAPPÉ

A quick note to my fellow non-meat eaters about the recipes:

Summer's menus can be adapted to suit everyone across the dietary spectrum. Her brilliant Meal Maps can be tweaked to include plant-based foods and her recipes can easily be adapted to your palate and preferences. *Bon appétit!*

Anna Lappé is a mom, sustainable food advocate, and best-selling author of three books, including *Diet for a Hot Planet: The Climate Crisis at the End of Your Fork,* and a contributing author to fifteen more. She is the founder and director of Real Food Media and works with philanthropists nationwide to help fund the grassroots change we need to create a healthier, more just, and sustainable food system.

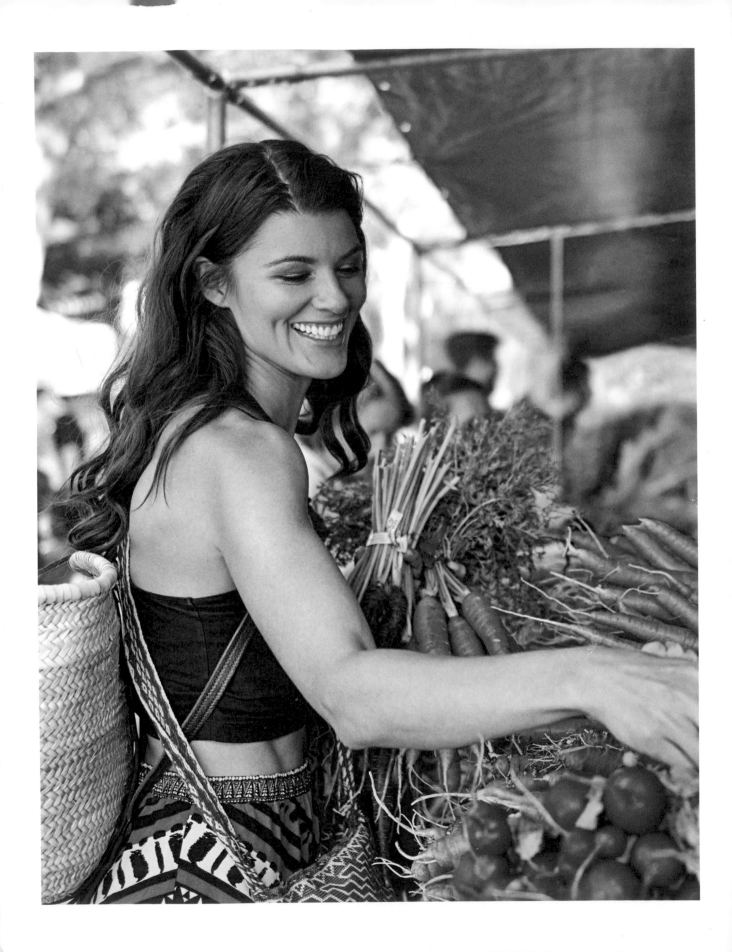

fidgeted restlessly on the piano seat. Pretty soon she took the attachment off the vacuum cleaner nozzle and began to remove the couch cushions. She started with the farthest cushion from the candy pile and began to vacuum the crevices—carefully rimming the corners of the sofa with its powerful suction. Then she removed the second cushion, placing it on top of the first on the coffee table. She cleaned every part thoroughly. My piano teacher walked through the kitchen. If only she would come out and start the piano lessons early! Her mother made a motion toward the last cushion, lifting it up in one fluid motion . . .

I played it off as if I didn't do it, but I *felt* and no doubt *looked* culpable. I was so mortified that I couldn't concentrate on my piano lesson—and clearly it's something I've never forgotten.

BLAME IT ON YOUR MOTHER . . . WELL, SORT OF

One day, when I was a little bit older, my mother admitted to me that she "craved sweet things" when she was pregnant with me. "I would eat bags and bags of oranges," she said. "I didn't have the same cravings when I was pregnant with your brother."

This was a revelation for me.

Although I didn't study for a degree in nutrition science, I am an environmental scientist by training, and I had a hunch that what my mom ate could have influenced my early childhood cravings. Taste preferences, as I found out, are indeed established in utero. It is projected that at 21 weeks after conception, growing fetuses begin gulping several ounces of amniotic fluid and, as a result, their smell and taste receptors are ignited. This amniotic fluid is flavored by what the mother eats. In fact, the sweeter it is, the more the baby wants to swallow.

By the time we are born, our taste is fairly developed, and it continues to develop, depending on what our mothers eat and whether we're fed breast milk or nursed on formula. The type of formula has an impact on a baby's preferences. Studies show that babies who are fed more bitter-tasting formulas will be more likely to prefer bitter foods as they mature. There is now evidence that those of us whose mothers ate more sugar before we were born have a higher likelihood of craving sugar, according to some peer-reviewed reports of animal trials. Those of us who might have been fed sweet fruits before vegetables might very well have a stronger preference for sweets, and, if we were particularly fussy babies, some of our mothers and fathers might not have had the patience, knowledge, or resources to try to feed us savory food at least thirteen times, which is the average number of times it usually take for a baby to accept a taste of something savory.

Our love of sugar goes even deeper than this. A recent study conducted on mice shows that mother mice with metabolic disorders can negatively affect three subsequent generations. Three generations! And don't think that your father or grandfather can get away scot-free, either. New evidence in rats shows that obesity and metabolic disorders can be passed from generation to generation through males, too. Scientists found that when babies were born, they were all in good metabolic health, but as soon as a high-fat, high-sugar, junk food diet was introduced, all the male rat offspring "reacted dramatically and within just a few weeks they developed fatty liver disease [and] pre-diabetic symptoms, such as elevated glucose and insulin in the bloodstream." And if both parents are compromised, you can assume a double whammy effect on their offspring. We're not rodents, but if this is any indication of what can happen to humans, we need to consider not only our health, but our kids' health, and their children's well-being.

The good news is that it's possible to curb your sweet tooth, as I've found out, and you can stop blaming your parents for it. More and more studies, both formal and informal, show that removing sugar from your diet, for even a short period of time—say two weeks—can reduce your taste for sugar. And rebalancing your brain with the proper vitamins, minerals, and amino acids will help reduce cravings so that you're set up for even more success! Eating is a learned behavior, and we are masters of our own destiny when it comes to our taste for food. And although it is true that some of us may have to contend with more challenging, uphill battles—for example, with leptin resistance, the "satiety hormone" that signals us to stop eating—or struggle with a high-stress lifestyle or the impact of having been exposed to too much fruit juice in utero, we can still put ourselves on a path to better health, when we have the curiosity and will to understand our body's needs and wants. The next step is reevaluating the way we live our life and exploring our personal cravings and relationship to food, as we all have our own unique story and experience to share. Then we can begin rediscovering the joy of eating well.

WHY I WROTE THIS BOOK

Given that so many of us can't seem to satisfy our sweet tooth, I felt compelled to create a web-based resource (SugarDetox.me) and this book to help you kick your sugar habit safely, easily, and effectively. At its very essence, *SugarDetoxMe* is a foundational guide and cookbook that will give you an achievable path toward better health. The book arms you with knowledge about what is happening to you when you eat sugar and suggests ways to change your behavior to help build the foundation of a healthier lifestyle. It also aims to reinvigorate your taste for food that is truly good for you, as well as simplify cooking to make healthy eating achievable for those of us who live busy lifestyles.

In order for a sugar cleanse to be effective, I realized that what is needed is not another fancy cookbook with impossibly complex recipes but, instead, an easy-to-follow, foolproof guide that offers healthy, affordable, and intuitive meals that are easy to make. The 100-plus recipes in this book are familiar, intuitive, easy, and non-fussy, and they contain ingredients that are affordable and readily available to most of us. The recipes are also designed to be flexible—so, if you add an extra quarter teaspoon of salt, or switch in kale for spinach, or use chicken broth instead of vegetable broth, don't hyperventilate! Your recipe will still work. This should come as a relief to those of us who aren't particularly well versed in the cooking department. The book will really give you an opportunity to feel much more confident in your abilities.

By the time you get to chapter 5, you'll discover Meal Maps, basic plans that list ingredients for a number of recipes and then show how those ingredients can be used across multiple meals in order to maximize your use of those ingredients, minimize waste, and help save money. Each Meal Map contains its own shopping list, recipe list, and meal plan to help you shop and eat better. Meal Maps are meant to be foundational, not rigidly prescriptive. In other words, feel free to swap out ingredients—like meat for beans or tempeh—or come up with your own Meal Maps. Have fun with the process, whatever you do. Meal Maps are meant to combine formulaic but versatile ways to make good food again and again, all while nixing sweet cravings, reducing the time you spend prepping and cooking food, and offering appetizing and energizing meals you'll enjoy.

What we eat is influenced by all sorts of internal and external cues. I encourage you to take a closer look at your own life so that you can achieve greater freedom from sugar. I'd like you to think of this book as a guide and a set of tools that will make healthy foods more inviting, accessible, and joy-ful! My hope is that *SugarDetoxMe* inspires you not only to reduce your sugar intake, but also to take your first step to making healthier overall lifestyle choices.

I encourage and invite you to take the time to explore your personal cravings and relationship to food, since none of us has the same story or experience. When you're able to put the pieces of your own puzzle together to see the whole picture, you'll begin to feel empowered to discover the path toward health!

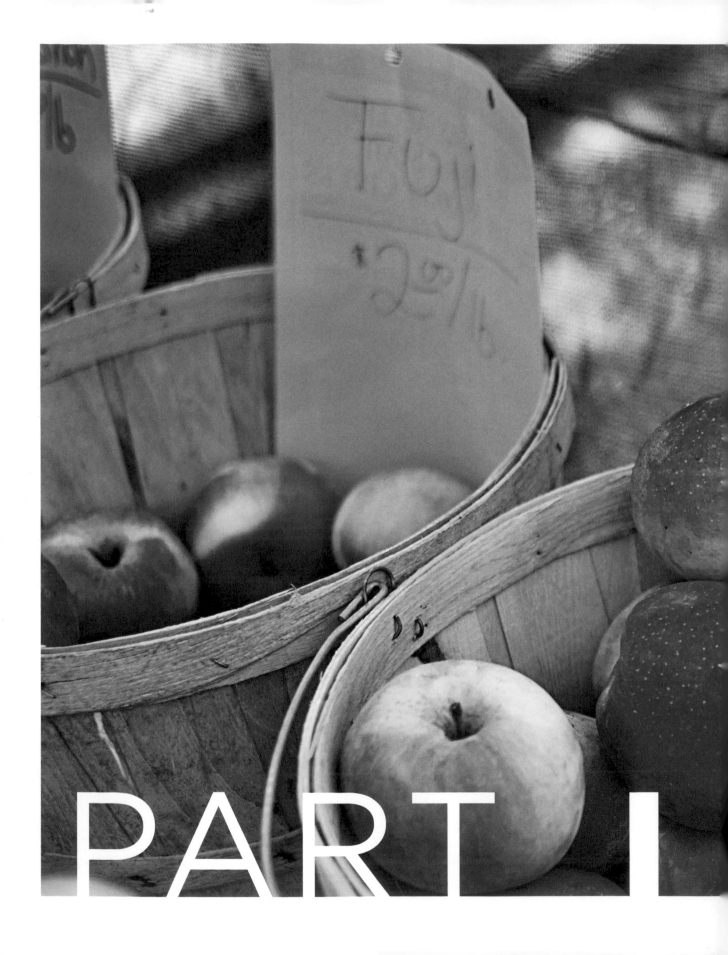

PART 1

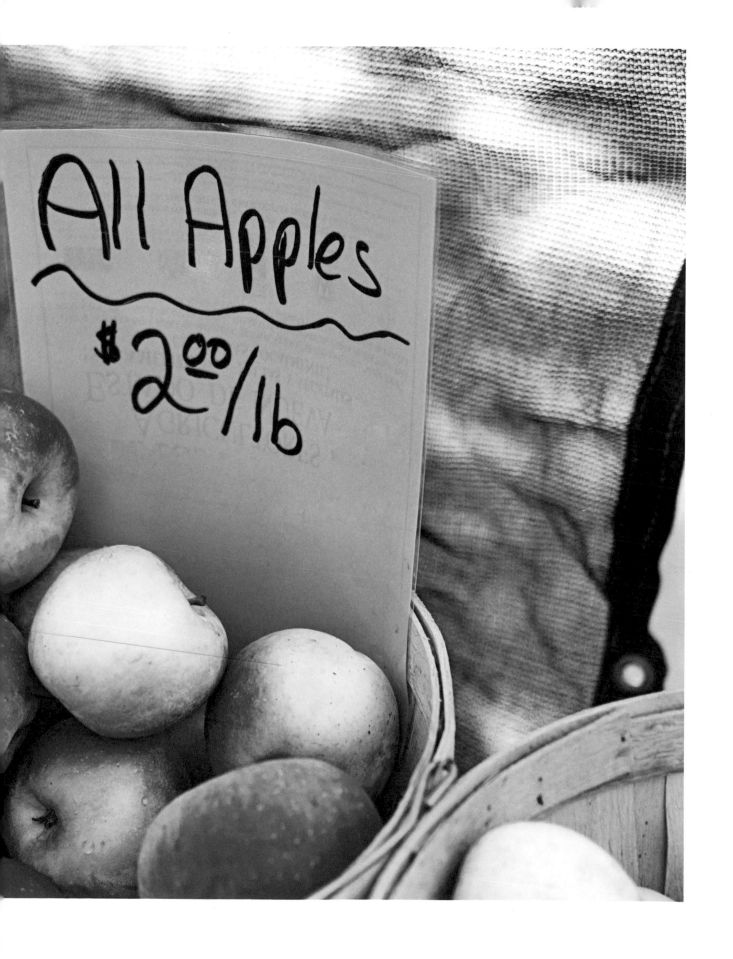

CHAPTER 1

WHY **DETOX** FROM SUGAR?

I'VE HAD A SWEET TOOTH FOR AS LONG AS I CAN REMEMBER. IF YOU HAVE ONE, TOO, I'M SURE YOU HAVE MORE THAN A FEW VIVID MEMORIES OF EATING—AND HOARDING—SWEET THINGS. I KNEW THERE WAS SOMETHING INHERENTLY WRONG ABOUT THIS WHEN I WAS GROWING UP, BUT I STILL FELT COMPELLED TO RAID THE COOKIE JAR, LITERALLY AND FIGURATIVELY.

Although not everyone struggles with a sweet tooth on a regular basis, we do have something in common: every single one of us is biologically hardwired to like sugar from the start, meaning we are programmed to want it even as infants. Mary Poppins, the acclaimed British nanny of the P. L. Travers books who was brought to life by Julie Andrews in Walt Disney's 1964 musical film, was onto something when she enthusiastically sang, "A spoonful of sugar helps the medicine go down!" But Poppins would blush to know that since the film was released, sugar consumption around the world has increased by more than 50 percent! Added sugar can now be found in everything from coffees to breads to sauces to cereals. Sugar's sweetness has the power to change your brain. As soon as a sugar molecule hits one of your tongue's 10,000 taste buds, a stimulus is shot off to your brain and gut, triggering your happiness centers and literally altering your biochemical pathways. If you do this enough times, your brain can become conditioned to want more and more sugar. This is because sugar can mimic and eventually replace or desensitize your natural feel-good neurotransmitters, which is why when you try to wean yourself off of sugar or quit it completely, you can get downright cranky. These are called abstinence symptoms, and they are just one of the many reasons why more scientists and people are looking at excessive sugar consumption as an addiction.

Sweetness receptors developed in the brains of our primate ancestors over 35 million years ago and carried over into humans. Carbohydrates, in the form of starches and sugars, provide glucose as energy for our bodies. It's that sweetness or starchiness that then triggers our reward centers. Sugar releases beta-endorphin, the chemical that produces the "runner's high," reducing pain and easing emotional distress. Dopamine, the "happy hormone," is released as well, and serotonin, the neurotransmitter found in our stomachs and brains that helps reduce anxiety and maintain overall mood, is elevated, too—at least temporarily.

In the past, food, including sugary substances, was scarcer and less available than it is now. In nature, highly concentrated sugars such as sugar cane, maple syrup, agave, and honey are extremely difficult and labor intensive to acquire—hiding behind woody stems, thick layers of bark and sapwood, hard spiny stalks, or stinging bees, respectively—a signal, perhaps, that this sugary sweetness should be savored once in a while, not cultivated and consumed daily. Now, we don't have to carry a hatchet or wear a bee suit to help us get to the sweet stuff without labor or injury; all we have to do is go to aisle 9 and get squeeze bottles filled with concentrated sugars. In fact, you can get a sugary dose from nearly eight out of ten products at the grocery store.

To compound the problem, we are far less active than people were even just one or two generations ago. My dad is a retired truck driver who worked on the docks, carrying and loading heavy boxes onto eighteen-wheelers; my mother is a retired dancer.

My grandparents and great grandparents were also quite active, working in construction, farming, and the coal mines of Pennsylvania. They worked hard so that we didn't have to labor in the same way. And they were successful! Now my brother (a computer engineer) and I (an entrepreneur-writer) spend 70 percent or more of our time sitting, along with the rest of our peers! A biological trigger to seek out starch and sugar makes sense if we were expending as much energy as my parents and grandparents, but we're sitting on our butts more of the time now yet still have that nagging biological trigger to want and crave sweetness.

WE "MEDICATE" OURSELVES WITH FOOD

We need to give the cells in our bodies the right nutrients in order to operate well over time. If we're not getting enough essential amino acids, vitamins, and minerals from our food, things tend to go wrong, and oftentimes we just don't listen to what our bodies are telling us. It's our amino acids—the essential and basic building blocks of protein—that turn into neurotransmitters in a process called methylation. If you have poor methylation (likely due to poor nutrition), then you'll have high homocysteine levels in your blood, which will no doubt set you up for cravings and even food addictions. Anyone who smokes, drinks a lot of coffee or other caffeinated beverages, drinks more than one glass of alcohol a day, or eats a lot of meat will additionally see a rise in homocysteine, which ultimately compounds sugar cravings and the effects of withdrawal, and burdens us with serious health risks over time.

But many of us do not eat for nutritional needs, but out of emotional ones. Boredom, anxiety, stress, and even fatigue can have us hitting the ice cream bowl. It's widely known that stress promotes poor diet, and let's face it: a lot of us are stressed and don't know how to deal with it. If you're constantly agitated at school or work, going through a difficult time, managing a bad breakup, or not getting enough sleep, no amount of willpower will keep you from buying those cookies if you're feeling imbalanced. If you can't get a handle on your stress, then you may have a more challenging if not impossible time cutting back on sugar, since sugar can make you feel better temporarily and ultimately override your healthy brain state. Sure, this book is primarily a cookbook, and you need to know which ingredients are preferable to eat and the best way to prepare them, but before we get to that, you'll need to do a close personal analysis into how you live your life on a daily basis and what you need to overcome first before even getting to the "tell me what to eat" part.

STEERING (YOUR SHOPPING CART) CLEAR OF SUGAR

Your emotions and how you live your life may be the most challenging aspect of all of this, but even if you do have a good handle on it all, there is another physical challenge. As soon as you decide to eat healthfully, you have to go find the good stuff and attempt to stave off what triggers you. Steering clear of the bagels and birthday cakes at the office or avoiding all but two or three aisles at a grocery store is tricky! Most of what you encounter at the supermarket is laced with sugar. Out of 600,000 food items in our nation's grocery stores, more than 75 percent contain added sugar. That's three out of four products!

There is now significantly compelling evidence that drinking sugary beverages, like soda, is causally related to increased risk of obesity and diabetes. This is due to a variety of reasons. First, if I were to ask you where digestion starts, I'd bet most people would say, "the stomach!" This is simply not true. Digestion starts in your mouth. Your appetite is reduced when you chew, driven by the nerves in your teeth to your brain. When you slurp down liquids, they aren't recognized by your nervous system and thus will leave you feeling hungry. Second, most smoothies and juices have little or no fiber content, respectively. It's fiber, particularly insoluble fiber, or intact "roughage" that helps aid digestion, keeps you satiated, and reduces sugar loads going into your body. This means after drinking liquids with "free" sugars (or sugar without the intact fiber), you tend to consume more, if not right away then likely later in the day. And finally, sugar in smoothie and juice drinks is often abnormally high, and with little or no fiber to slow sugar uptake in your body, it ends up taxing your liver and changing the biochemistry of your brain.

People are picking up on this more and more. Just as I was finishing the first draft of this book, I passed two ladies on Bedford Avenue in Brooklyn, New York. "Have some orange juice," the one on the left insisted, holding out a large bottle of freshly squeezed juice.

"Nooooo," the woman on the right replied in a most irritated manner. "It's got so much sugar!"

"But it's *only* orange juice," the first woman retorted, as she walked by me.

I'm sure her friend, who refused the juice, taught her something about sugar that day.

If you take only one thing away from this book that will immediately benefit your health, I would suggest cutting out all sugary drinks, including sodas, sports drinks, energy drinks, sweetened teas and coffees, fruit juices, fresh pressed fruit juices, smoothies, and certain kinds of alcohol.

As Marion Nestle, a New York University professor of sociology, points out in her book *Soda Politics: Taking on Big Soda (and Winning)*, sugary beverages account for half of all sugars consumed in the United States. Consumption of sodas alone accounts for one-third of that caloric intake. That's a huge amount! The American Beverage Association reported that Americans spent a total of $65 billion on soda in 2012—about six times more than what we spend on water and approximately the same amount that the United States spends on discretionary funding for education programs for our kids! That's a lot of money for a can of sugar, caffeine, and water. That's why if you're going to do one thing for yourself, you should drop the soda and sugary drinks. It's only going to benefit you.

Even though sodas account for a third of our calories, a determinant for good health is not really about the calories, despite what we've been told—which is part of the reason why you won't find any calorie-counting in this book. Determinants for good health are keeping your homocysteine levels low, insulin in check, and fructose levels within reason.

Glucose, a simple sugar, is an important energy source in every living being. Every cell in your body can metabolize it, which is why if you eat food that is high in glucose, it'll raise your blood sugar and trigger your pancreas to produce insulin to shuttle it out of your system, either turning it into energy for your body or storing it in your muscles or fat for later use. It's the reason why diabetics are told to watch their glycemic index (GI) and glycemic load (GL). Glucose can become chronically toxic if your body can't maintain it within the normal range, as in diabetes. Otherwise, all cells use it as an energy source.

Fructose, another simple sugar, can be found naturally in fruits and vegetables (often with the fiber intact!), or it can be synthesized and/or concentrated in table sugar, high fructose corn syrup, and fruit juices. Generally, fructose is metabolized only in your liver. If you eat enough of it (often the case!), it can be converted to fat, ultimately taxing your liver and your body, which is why fructose is now beginning to be considered a chronic liver toxin. It can also trigger insulin resistance. As Leslie Lee, a registered dietician and director of education and community engagement at the Institute for Responsible Nutrition, explained to me, "Fructose exerts no direct effect on insulin immediately following its consumption. However, fructose has an indirect, positive effect on insulin in the long term. After consumption, excess fructose is converted to fat in the liver. Some of that fat gets deposited in the liver, and when that happens, the liver becomes insulin resistant. When the liver is insulin resistant, the pancreas has to produce more insulin to overcome the resistance. So fructose indirectly raises insulin over time. An elevated insulin level then triggers weight gain and prevents the breakdown of fat between meals to be used as energy." In addition to this, doctors have begun to realize that elevated fructose in the body over time could lower circulating leptin—the satiety hormone that basically tells your body, 'I'm full now!"—and induce impaired glucose tolerance, hypertension, and other metabolic disorders.

The World Health Organization has released a frightening report in which it is revealed that one in 11 adults throughout the world are now diabetic, a quadrupling since I was born. And in California alone, it is estimated that over half of the adults (55%) in the state are either prediabetic or diabetic, with one-third of young adults (18–39 years old) having prediabetes. This disproportionately affects people of color, too, and it's very much linked to our food. An early study showed that foreign-born blacks have lower infant mortality than native-born blacks, likely due to better nutrition and less stress.

Type 2 diabetes used to be referred to as "adult-onset diabetes" because it was traditionally confined to a disease that parents—or grandparents—would get, not children. My mother used to seriously chide me when I would grab a handful of sweets at my grandparents' house: "If you eat that, you can get diabetes," she'd say with a look of worry. It almost became a joke to me because she'd say it so often—sort of like the boy who cried wolf. Little did I know, my mother was a clairvoyant. Though I skirted diabetes in my own life, that's not the case for a quarter of teenagers in the United States. Now, nearly one in four teens has diabetes or is prediabetic, the term for the precursor stage to diabetes mellitus, in which one's blood sugar is abnormally high.

A recent Credit Suisse report reveals that 90 percent of physicians across the United States, Europe, and Asia view dietary sugars as the cause of diabetes. Excessive sugar consumption can also lead to obesity in less direct ways. We now know that sugar changes our brain, affecting our biochemical pathways and our hormone signaling. It may make us feel hungrier or never satiated, compelling us to eat more sugar and more food in general, which can lead to obesity, which can be defined simply as a defect in which our bodies store energy.

Currently more than one-third of adults in America are obese, and childhood obesity (ages 2 to 19) has more than tripled and quadrupled in teens since the early '80s—or for as long as I have been alive. We live in a country where one out of three children and adolescents are overweight or obese, where obesity has become the number one greatest health concern for parents over drug abuse, smoking, and gun violence, and where diabetes is expected to afflict one in three Americans by 2050.

These are sobering facts!

It would be tempting to consider this a disease or epidemic, but it's more of a symptom of an unhealthy, imbalanced food system. Read: bad food is the epidemic. Being obese or, in some cases, overweight can increase your chances of being ill, but even then, it's not always that cut and dried. Some studies show that up to 40 percent of "normal" weight people have metabolic dysfunctions, too, including diabetes, hypertension, and cardiovascular disease. And around 20 percent of obese people do not have any of these conditions and go on to live perfectly healthy, normal lives. If one's obesity is diet-related, having access to and eating real, unprocessed food can help curb health risks. A recent study done by Dr. Robert Lustig, professor of pediatrics in the Division of Endocrinology at the University of California, San Francisco, and colleagues reported in the *New York Times* that obese children who replaced sugar intake with starches saw improvements in their blood pressure, cholesterol readings, and other health markers after just 10 days, which is something we do with the guided sugar cleanses on SugarDetox.me.

All of this is very promising, but changing our diets takes more than convincing ourselves that some food is bad and that we shouldn't eat it. We know that certain food is a "no-no," that we should refrain from indulging, but we haven't stopped. Why is that? It's because this is something that can't be solved with just information and logic. When we have an addiction or even a dependence on sugar, it's not the logical part of our brain that's affected; it's the limbic system of our brain, which controls instinct, mood, and habit.

According to Abigail Carroll, a food historian and author of *Three Squares: The Invention of the American Meal,* we make approximately 200 food choices every day, and most of them are done on autopilot. Knowledge is power, but since eating is a learned behavior and, in many cases, habitual, real change occurs by first learning to pay attention to our eating habits and second by removing barriers, whether they are biological (e.g., "My body is compelling me to eat!"), systemic (e.g., "Oh, our whole food system is out of whack!"), psychological (e.g., "I'll always be like this), cultural (e.g., "My family has been drinking soda for years!"), or economic (e.g., "There is nowhere I can get fresh, healthy food—and even if I could, I wouldn't be able to afford it."). Some or all of these barriers may afflict us, and it's important to recognize how to address them and utterly surround ourselves in healthier environments, practices, and routines, whether that means working on our sleep hygiene or clearing our kitchen shelves of trigger foods.

If anything, the good news in all of this is that once we identify the barriers, our food habits are adaptable, and we can reignite our pleasure in healthy food. We just have to work at it and give ourselves a chance to like what "healthy" really tastes like, and build better habits. The information, recipes, and meal plans in this book (and the corresponding online program), therefore, shouldn't be viewed as a short-term diet, but instead as something that helps us understand how to rebalance our brains and learn how to incorporate what we eat into a healthier lifestyle. This may mean we have to work at it consciously and regularly until it becomes quite simply how we live our lives.

CHAPTER 2

YOUR SUGAR **DETOX** GUIDE

BEFORE YOU BEGIN

IF YOU ARE MAKING A RADICAL OR SUBSTANTIAL CHANGE TO YOUR DIET, I STRONGLY RECOMMEND THAT YOU CONSULT WITH YOUR PHYSICIAN, REGISTERED DIETITIAN, OR HOLISTIC PRACTITIONER. EVEN THOUGH REMOVING EXCESS SUGARS, ALBEIT GRADUALLY, IS MORE THAN LIKELY TO BE A POSITIVE MOVE FOR MOST OF US, YOU MAY HAVE PRECONDITIONS THAT WILL MAKE IT A CHALLENGE, OR EVEN NEXT TO IMPOSSIBLE, TO ACCOMPLISH. FOR INSTANCE, IF YOU ARE DIABETIC, YOU NEED TO MANAGE YOUR BLOOD SUGAR LEVELS APPROPRIATELY. IF YOU HAVE ANOREXIA OR ANY OTHER SERIOUS EATING DISORDER, I ADVISE YOU TO SPEAK WITH YOUR DOCTOR OR AN EATING-DISORDER PROFESSIONAL FOR GUIDANCE AND A PLAN THAT IS RIGHT FOR YOU IN PARTICULAR. ADDITIONALLY, IF YOU HAVE NEUROCHEMICAL AND HORMONAL IMBALANCES—LIKE LOW SEROTONIN LEVELS OR LEPTIN RESISTANCE—THOSE IMBALANCES MUST BE APPROPRIATELY ADDRESSED BEFORE CHANGING YOUR EATING HABITS.

Everyone's body is different, and the condition of our bodies differs vastly, too—even on a day-to-day basis. If you are running on four hours of sleep every night or waking up every couple of hours to nurse or put your baby back to bed, you'll likely be stressing your body, which will give you more food cravings. If this is part of your lifestyle, it's important to acknowledge and plan around it so that you don't find yourself scarfing down whatever is available to you whenever you feel stressed. I cannot emphasize enough how important a role good overall health—like sleep hygiene and a positive attitude—plays in the success of a sugar cleanse.

That brings me to my next point. If you have made a commitment to yourself to do a sugar detox, stay positive. Psych yourself up! I prepared myself psychologically for six months before I started my own sugar detox, because I wanted to feel empowered with all the information that was available to me. Then I put together a ten-step program for myself that I knew I could follow, which I'll share with you. Even if I slipped up down the road (totally normal!), I knew I had a reliable framework that I could come back to again and again. So if you slip up for whatever reason, don't beat up on yourself. Practice some self-love first.

GETTING STARTED ON YOUR JOURNEY

If any of you are like me, at some point you may have realized, "Whoa, I probably need to cut back on my sugar intake!" I always had a sweet tooth and didn't really make the time to figure out why it was afflicting me and how to cut back successfully until relatively recently.

Knowing how sugar and, more specifically, fructose was affecting my body and tricking my system into wanting it really helped me understand what type of framework I needed to follow for my own success. And I should say now that it's important to define what "success" is for you over a period of time. Give yourself as long as you need to psychologically prepare yourself for your sugar cleanse journey and *at least* a month (but preferably three months) of eating well in the spirit of this book. In ten days, you'll likely see or feel positive results, if not sooner. Some people who do as little as a week of cleansing with me see great results within a few days, from energy gains to weight loss.

Of course, removing added sugars from your diet can also have other seemingly adverse reactions called abstinence symptoms, including headaches, energy dips, and intense cravings. You may become a very, very grumpy person. These withdrawal symptoms are totally normal. And they suck. Big time. They happen because our blood sugar takes some time to stabilize and our brain needs a chance to reboot, which means producing its own neurotransmitters again, fueled by healthy foods rich in amino acids, vitamins, and minerals. This is just part of the reason why sugar is now starting to be classified by some scientists and health professionals as an addictive substance. If you've tried to rid yourself of caffeine or other addictive substances, like alcohol, you'll soon realize that this is normal, and you'll likely get past it, if you have patience and adequate contingency plans, like taking vitamin, mineral, and amino acid supplements to help give your body a healthy jump-start. It's just one of the reasons why this book *isn't* considered a "diet book." You're simply removing a substance that, when eaten in excess, can be a chronic toxin to your body. And removing toxins is *not* a diet.

What this process will do is help put your overall health front and center, while allowing you to take a look at other aspects of your life that may contribute to your cravings. It also sets you up with the tools, skills, and confidence to go forward with the idea of establishing or reestablishing a healthy diet. Once you have your health, which is arguably the most important aspect of anyone's life, you'll find that it will trickle into other parts of your life. You may want to start exercising more. You may want to go out with friends. You might even want to dress up. Heck, you might even want to start posting your healthy food on your Instagram feed to share your good meals with everyone (just be sure to include #sugardetoxme on those posts so I can find them)!

THE IMPORTANCE OF STAYING MIND AND BODY POSITIVE

On a personal note, I think one of the most important aspects of going on a sugar cleanse, or doing anything else, for that matter, is staying mind and body positive. Coming from the world of fashion, as a model, and also as a woman, I am acutely aware of how much we are bombarded every day with unrealistic images of bodies, and unrealistic demands and expectations.

One day at the gym I was approached by a beautiful, vibrant, and physically fit forty-year-old woman who admitted that she had some body image issues. She had noticed that I never weighed myself and never looked obsessively in the mirror or at other people's bodies. She asked how I had developed—at least in her eyes—a healthy approach to my body. When I go to the gym or go for a run, I don't do it with the goal of whittling down my waist or trimming my tush—I go with the idea that I *love* to feel my body move. I like the way it feels when I'm able to pick up a good stride, or feel euphoria when I dance, or get into a good stretch. You can get that feeling, regardless of your shape or size. I put the emphasis on the part that is fun, and if my waist and tush get trimmer because of it, then so be it. That, in my opinion, is a healthy approach to life, and one that we should bring to our relationship to food, as well.

No one wants to pay for something—whether it's a meal at a restaurant, a fashion magazine, or a gym membership—only to feel belittled, guilty, or ostracized. On the contrary, we want to do things that make us feel included, inspired, and supported. This guide and cookbook is all about that—so consider it your source of positive motivation! And even though I'll be going over the food that you should avoid on a sugar detox, the idea is to really focus on the delicious foods that you will be eating. You'll get back into the joy of cooking and training your body to seek out different flavor profiles and full nutrition so that you can give your body and mind more of what they need. So let's focus less on abstinence and more on sustenance!

NOTE: *See The Wheel of Life Exercise, a powerful visualization tool that can help you come to terms with your sugar tooth and bring your life back in balance, in Appendix A, on page 241.*

THE FOUR GOALS OF THIS SUGAR DETOX AND COOKBOOK

It's easy to focus on—or should I say villainize—one ingredient, and even though you are concentrating on reducing sugar in your diet over the short and long terms, I want to emphasize that this book and program are based on four underpinning goals:

Developing a no-stress, healthy approach to eating—one that will last a lifetime!

Placing more importance on health, and the happiness that stems from being healthy.

Developing an ability to listen more closely to your body.

Ultimately gaining the knowledge, skills, and routine to make eating whole, healthy, and healing foods a reality—without all that sugar.

WHAT IS SUGAR ANYWAY, AND WHY IS IT SO BAD FOR YOU?

Sugars are not inherently bad for you, but they can affect your personal genetic makeup and have a damaging affect on your health, depending on which sugars you consume and how much and how often you consume them. When sugar is used in foodstuffs, it is often disguised by at least five dozen different names, from high fructose corn syrup (HFCS) to agave. (See Appendix C, page 251, for a full list.) This masquerade is part of the food industry's strategy to confuse you about what you're actually eating. In addition to this, labels may also list one of several sugar alcohols, such as erythritol and xylitol, as well as alternative sweeteners, such as aspartame, monk fruit, and more—all of which will loosely be referred to as "sugars" for ease and simplicity in this book.

SUGAR BY ANY OTHER NAME

Throughout this book "sugar" is used as a general term for a sweetened substance. Here you'll find definitions for some of the most used terms for sugar and the differences between them.

Natural sugars: Sugars that occur naturally in foods, such as whole beets or whole fruits, like apples, oranges, and milk.

Added sugars: Sugars, syrups, and artificial sweeteners that are added to foods or beverages when they are processed or prepared. Added sugars (also called added sweeteners) include natural sugars (such as white sugar, brown sugar, dates, fruit juice, maple syrup, and honey) and chemically manufactured sweeteners (such as high fructose corn syrup).

Free sugars: Sugar that is simply unbound by fiber. Free sugars are inclusive of added sugars and can also exist naturally, like honey or maple syrup, or it can result from the removal or obliteration of fiber, such as in juicing or blending.

Alternative sugars: Food additives, produced either naturally or synthetically, that provide a sweet taste like that of sugar. They are also known as sugar substitutes. Those produced synthetically are also called artificial sweeteners.

Sugar alcohols: Organic compounds derived from sugars. They typically have low sweetness, so they are often used in combination with alternative sugars. They are a good alternative to sugar because they do not promote tooth decay, but they can still affect blood sugar levels. They are often marketed in "sugar-free" products.

HOW LITTLE SUGAR IS RECOMMENDED IN OUR DIETS?

According to the World Health Organization, the 2015 Dietary Guidelines Advisory Committee, and the National Health Service in the United Kingdom, it's advisable to keep free sugar intake below 10 percent of our total energy (or caloric) intake, and if you're already on your way to a sugar-related disease, it should be below 5 percent. This could be a little misleading though, since counting calories is not always the best way to monitor intake, as all calories are not created equal, but guidelines are there to serve as guideposts.

So what does 10 percent or 5 percent of our total energy intake mean? Well, if you are counting calories and have a 2,000 calorie diet per day, then you should be having no more than 200 calories or 100 calories, respectively, coming from added sugar. One hundred calories from sugar, is around 8 small squares from your favorite 70% dark chocolate bar. Not much, right?! And if you want to understand this better, 1 teaspoon of sugar is roughly 16 calories. Another way of looking at it is through teaspoons and grams. According to the American Heart Association, women should have no more than 6 teaspoons (about 25 grams) of added sugar per day, and men should have no more than 9 teaspoons (37.5 grams). The average American, however actually consumes closer to 22 teaspoons per day (92.4 grams), while Australians consume up to 27 teaspoons per day (113.4 grams), and Britons are taking in 14 teaspoons (58.8 grams)—all without even realizing it. So let's revisit your favorite dark chocolate bar. If four squares of dark chocolate contain 12 grams of sugar, that's about 3 teaspoons of sugar, which is equivalent to 48 calories (3 teaspoons sugar x 16 calories/teaspoon = 48 calories of sugar). That's half of the daily free sugar allowance suggested for a woman!

. . . .

SUGAR CONVERSION CHART

1 teaspoon sugar = 4.2 grams = 16 calories

RECOMMENDED UPPER LIMIT OF SUGAR CONSUMPTION BY AGE*

2–3 years: 4 teaspoons / 16.8 grams sugar

4–8 years: 3 teaspoons / 12.6 grams sugar

9–18 years: 5–8 teaspoons / 21–33.6 grams sugar

19+ years: 6–9 teaspoons / 25.2–37.8 grams sugar

*The number ranges denote the upper limit for females (lower end) and males (higher end).

HOOKED ON JUICE?

I was in the grocery store recently and took a walk down the juice and sugary beverage aisle. There you can find everything from sports drinks to "all-natural" juices. Well, clearly the blue sports drink is "unnatural" and the cranberry juices are "natural," right? Not so fast! In many cases, that cranberry, apple, or orange juice—even if it's "unsweetened"—can have more than 30 grams of sugar in one serving, or 1 cup, of juice. The fact that the fruit has been juiced and the natural sugar has been concentrated without any corresponding fiber makes this free sugar, unbound by fiber, and it will undoubtedly give your body a sharp sugar spike, particularly if you're drinking it alone, without any fibrous food. We shouldn't be eating sugar—natural or otherwise—in excess; there is absolutely no need for free sugars in our diet, since they do not serve any nutritive or physiological purpose. They can be useful to provide quick energy, but our bodies can produce glucose through noncarbohydrate sources, such as proteins, through an entirely different metabolic pathway.

That's why you'll notice that there aren't any juice or smoothie recipes in this book. Quite frankly, many fruit-based and some veggie-based juices and smoothies have way too much free sugar. Evidence from the National Health Service in the United Kingdom and leading-edge scientists show that sugar found in fruit juices and smoothies, which are naturally occurring, should definitely be restricted. The sugar that would have otherwise been contained within the structure of whole fruit is released when the fruit is juiced or partially obliterated when blended. In the case of smoothies, the soluble fiber is still there, but the insoluble fiber matrix will have been blended to smithereens.

A 1977 study by Haber et al. showcases this effect. Even though the study was small, the results were statistically significant and conclusive: The blood glucose and insulin response to whole apples was increased by blending the apples to a puree (smoothie) and by extracting the juice (juicing) and there was a "striking rebound fall [of the plasma glucose] after juice and to a lesser extent after the puree," which was not seen after the consumption of the whole apples. Serum insulin then rose to higher levels for both juice and puree, so the study concluded that yes, when making juices or smoothies, you are definitely disturbing your glucose balance largely due to fiber loss or destruction of the fiber matrix.

It also should be pointed out that juices and smoothies in general usually contain way more than the two servings of whole fruit per day that we should be aiming for in our diets. *The NY Daily News* recently revealed the amount of sugar in some popular juice cleanses, which have become all the rage for a lot of my friends. They range from 75 grams of sugar per day (50 grams over the suggested daily limit for women) to 146–191 grams of sugar per day. The latter is like drinking the equivalent of three to five cans of soda per day. It's a sugar bomb to the bloodstream! The National Health Service says 100 percent fruit juice is still a healthy choice, particularly if you're not getting your daily intake of whole fruits and veggies, but if you are going to drink your juice, then I would suggest drinking water first, and then drink the juice along with a meal, and have no more than one serving a day, which is around 150 milliliters or just a little over 1 cup.

HOW SUGAR AFFECTS YOUR BODY

Have you ever wondered why sugar has become increasingly prominent in virtually every packaged or prepared food we eat? Sugar, by no fault of its own, was designed to not only taste good but also reward our biochemical pathways, releasing neurotransmitters like beta-endorphin and dopamine. Because of that, sugar can override self-control mechanisms and prompt you to eat more of it. Food executives looking to get customers hooked would quickly realize that they could do so legally with a generous dose of sugar. Michael Moss, the author of *Salt, Sugar, Fat: How the Food Giants Hooked Us*, writes, "the optimum amount of sugar in a product became known as the 'bliss point,'" and food inventors are obsessed with finding the exact amount that keeps us coming back for more. He reports that some of the largest food companies have been employing the use of brain scans to understand how we neurologically respond to sugar (it's not unlike how our brains would respond to cocaine, another highly addictive and harmful substance). As a matter of fact—at least in rat studies—sugar is far more addictive than cocaine. A 2007 report demonstrated that when given the option of water sweetened with saccharin or intravenous cocaine, 94 percent of rats preferred the sweet taste of saccharin. Increasing the doses of cocaine didn't even override the preference for sugar in the rats.

Some scientists struggle with whether to consider sugar addictive, but more compelling evidence is emerging to show addictive behaviors in many of us. As a result, we're starting to see the emergence of the first sugar addiction programs. Not surprisingly, any substance that causes us to compulsively want it is compelling to big business. According to a recent report from BCC Research, the global market share for sugar and sweeteners in 2012 was $77.5 billion and is projected to grow to around $97 billion by the time this book comes out.

Refined sugars were virtually absent in our diets for much of human history, so it should come as no surprise that our bodies aren't used to the chemical assault that we have unleashed upon them. Three hundred years ago people in Europe on average consumed a measly 4 pounds per year! This was in part due to the novelty of sugar and its hefty price tag. During that time a pound of sugar cost the equivalent of around $45 in today's dollars, which is far pricier than the $0.65 per pound it costs at retail now. Today in America, we're on average consuming around 1.45 pounds per week, or around 76 pounds per year. Just imagine—76 pounds per year and 300 years ago we were consuming a measly 4 pounds annually! After learning more about what we're doing to our bodies and reflecting on my past obsession with sugar, I began to feel more empowered and energized to make a change—and I know you will, too.

10 STEPS TO SUGAR **DETOX**

When I first decided to do a sugar cleanse to see if I could reduce or even eliminate my cravings, I did it with the idea that I would come up with a framework that would help me succeed. What could I do to keep honest, un-tempted, and on course? I began to jot down the process I was already doing naturally, which involved first learning as much as possible about the topic. This empowered me and eventually led to the creation of the 10 steps below. They are just examples of some of the actions you can take; let them serve as a guide, but also keep your mind open to other techniques that might help you as you navigate your own sugar detox journey.

STEP 1. Know That Food Addiction and Food Dependence Is Real

The concept of a food addiction or food dependence is relatively new—so new that we're just starting to see the first sugar and carbohydrate addiction clinics emerging. In the past, if I saw someone who was morbidly obese or eating their fifth candy bar, I would think to myself that she or he had a lack of willpower or discipline—a common assumption. However, it's simply not true. More than 10 years ago, Richard L. Atkinson, emeritus professor of medicine and nutritional science at the University of Wisconsin, wrote in the journal *Nutrition and Health* that this assumption is no longer defensible, given all the current studies that show how sugar and other substances definitively alter our biochemical pathways and release opioids and dopamine. The takeaway is that sugar literally impacts your behavior.

This statement is an absolute paradigm shift in the way we think about what we eat and why we eat it. Atkinson's assessment is easy to see, however, once you understand how sugar manipulates your mind, leading to very clear behavior and neurochemical changes. Studies, particularly in animal trials but also observed in humans, show bingeing, withdrawal, craving, and cross-sensitization, which refers to a phenomenon in which a person becomes sensitized to other substances (like amphetamine), with sugar as the instigator. These behaviors relate to neurochemical changes in the brain, something that also happens with addictive drugs. This varies, however, from person to person, so we have to be careful: just because a food addiction or food dependence exists, it doesn't mean we all have one. And what we eat, why we eat, when we eat, and how we eat are also influenced by many internal and external factors, from our friends to food marketing. In short, food is personal on many levels. Some of us may self-medicate with food, particularly with sugar, but not all of us do. As you go through these steps and begin to understand how sugar affects your behavior, you'll be able to focus more clearly on what you're feeling when a craving arises.

STEP 2. Learn How Biochemical Pathways in Your Body Change When You Eat Sugar

Did you ever say, "I just feel it in my gut," when something feels off or you feel a little creeped out? There is a good reason for that. You're likely more in tune with your body, because your bowels are literally dubbed "the second brain." It turns out that we have a mass of neural tissue in our gut called the enteric nervous system. This "brain" in your belly contains more than 100 million neurons and more than 30 neurotransmitters. It's 1/100th fewer than the neurons in your brain, but it's still quite a lot. These are used to communicate back and forth, so your brain-gut connection is a strong one. In fact, 95 percent of the body's serotonin is found in the gut. Serotonin mellows us out. It likely evolved because we generally eat when we feel safe, and your stomach sends you the signal to eat only when you feel secure. When you eat, it's a comfort. If you've ever taken antidepressant pills (or filled up on refined carbs, sugar, alcohol, and white bread) to raise your serotonin levels, it may have resulted in some gastrointestinal complications or upset, largely because it's triggering the serotonin production in your stomach.

Endorphins are often also released when you eat sweets, starches, and fats. These help relieve discomfort and pain and allow you to temporarily feel good. If you eat sugar, beta-endorphin is released, and you'll likely want to eat more sugar, which will release more beta-endorphin, which makes you want to eat even more. Stress triggers the release of dynorphin, a type of endorphin that is a powerful appetite stimulant. When you eat, the act of chewing releases dopamine, and dopamine comforts. In short, stress is comforted by eating. Sugar dependents often turn to sugars and starches for comfort. When you eat sugar, your dopamine levels—or reward centers—are turned on, making you feel good. The problem? Over time, you become desensitized and need to eat more and more sugar to obtain that same level of dopamine release. And of course, when insulin is released, it shuttles the sugar out of your blood, and you hit a low again until you are able to get your next "hit" of sugar.

STEP 3. Find Out If You Have a Food Dependence or Addiction

Since the idea of food dependence or food addiction is relatively new and still a bit controversial, there has been a dearth of measurement tools in the area. This all changed, however, when Ashley Gearhardt and colleagues at the Yale's Rudd Center for Food Policy and Obesity produced the Yale Food Addiction Scale (YFAS) in 2009. The scale included 25 questions designed to identify whether someone has a dependence on high-fat and high-sugar foods. Gearhardt, who is now an assistant professor in the Department of Psychology at the University of Michigan, became interested in food dependencies when she was researching alcohol addiction. "I've always been interested in what compels us to do one thing when we know we should be doing another," she shared over the phone. "Addiction is an extreme version of this. A person who is addicted wants to stop but can't. Why is that?" That very question has guided her subsequent studies.

In 2009, the YFAS was updated to include a series of 35 questions, in order to maintain consistency with the

Diagnostic and Statistical Manual of Mental Disorders (5th ed.; *DSM-5*), making it the most up-to-date measurement of addiction when it comes to food.

But even with this tool, Gearhardt explains, there are complications and sometimes more questions than answers. "Within the world of addiction, there is so much heterogeneity [diversity]," she says. "Food affects the brain differently than say alcohol. Food doesn't go past the blood-brain barrier—but then again," she points out, " neither does gambling," which was upgraded from an impulse-control disorder to an addiction in May 2013. And there are many more variables when it comes to the food we eat. "In our culture, there is such an emphasis on dieting and looking a certain way. You have to begin to disentangle all of those psychological effects," Gearhardt says. "We are just now trying to uncover those complexities."

Thanks to Gearhardt's work, however, we now have a framework in which to self-analyze our own eating habits in ways that, perhaps, we haven't given much thought to before.

To use the Yale Food Addiction Survey (YFAS), refer to Appendix B on page 243.

STEP 4. Know Where Sugar Comes From

On average, nearly half of our sugar intake comes from sugary beverages, like soda, sports drinks, and fruit juices. Prepared foods (ketchup, spreads, canned vegetables and fruits), grain-based desserts, dairy-based desserts, and cereals also add unnecessary sugar to our diets.

Different people get their sugar from different foods, so it's a good idea to keep a food journal, at least for the first month of your sugar detox, so that you can be more mindful of what you're actually eating, when you're eating it, and why you're eating it. Self-monitoring, though it may become a tedious task over the long run, helps you become far more aware of what triggers you in the moment, keeps you in check with portion-control, helps you stay focused on long-term progress, and, if done digitally, allows you to track progress easily over time.

There are a lot of ways to keep a food diary, from using just a pen and paper to a variety of monitoring apps. No matter what tool you use, self-monitoring can help you lose weight, if that is your goal. Tools that are technologically based—like an app or even a memo on your phone—can help you be more consistent when you record information. For me, a Google doc or electronic memo pad works best, since I don't particularly like to use tracking apps.

KEEPING A FOOD JOURNAL

Make your food journal as detailed as possible:

1. **What** food you eat

2. **How much** food you're eating

3. **How many** carbohydrates and sugars (and fiber, if possible!)

4. **What time** of day you're eating

5. **Where** you are when you're eating

6. **How you feel** at the moment when you're eating

7. **What you are doing** (if anything) while you are eating

Here are some examples of what your entries might look like:

1. Brand X popcorn

2. 1 bag, 18 grams

3. 13 grams of carbs in one bag, 3 grams of sugar

4. 3 p.m.

5. At work

6. Feeling bored—that midday, after lunch slump!

7. Working at my computer

My hunch is that once you start to record for a week, 2 weeks, 1 month or more, you'll start to see some noticeable eating habits emerge. "Hmmm," you may say. "I see that I eat at my desk whenever I'm bored." From there, you can begin making behavioral shifts. Perhaps eating popcorn has become an accidentally conditioned behavior, meaning it's just a temporary diversion from your boredom, rewarding you for sitting diligently at your desk all day. Instead, see if you can reward yourself by chatting with a colleague, taking a walk down the block, or even closing your computer for a few moments to go look out the window. If you think it's actual hunger that's making you get up and not boredom, then come up with a healthier snack, like a package of raw almonds or a whole fruit.

STEP 5. Research the Best Foods to Eat

There are so many ways to go about a sugar cleanse, so, it really depends on what is right for you. When I did mine, I decided to remove all free sugars, or sugars unbound from fiber; processed starches, like white bread, pasta, and white rice; and most sugary fruits and vegetables, like dates and beets, from my diet for at least 30 days. It was a way for me to do a nutritional reset and evaluate more fully how I felt when those ingredients weren't a part of my diet. I was psychologically and physically prepared to do the cleanse, and pumped to make the time to commit to it.

For folks who also have a clear addiction to sugary substances (which is a good reason to see where you fall on the YFAS, on page 243), nutritionists will often recommend quitting trigger ingredients and foods cold turkey. The same principle applies to an alcohol or drug addiction: "Have only one drink" is almost like an open invite to have two, three, four, or more—particularly if you're feeling down. It's hard to quit. Dealing with the emotions and symptoms of withdrawal is undoubtedly tough, but going through it with a plan will give you the skills and eventually the confidence to overcome anything.

You might want to take a more gradual, incremental route, however, rather than go cold turkey—and behavioral science shows that this can help you develop better eating habits over the long-run. There is a smart way to do this: first by removing sugary beverages, then by removing other food products that contain free sugars, and then replacing refined carbohydrates altogether. Additionally, you can talk to a nutritionist, a nutritional therapist, or your health practitioner about whether you can and should take any nutritional supplements, such as amino acids, vitamins, and minerals, to help alleviate any withdrawal symptoms. Typical supplements that nutritionists may suggest include omega-3s, tryptophan or 5HTP, B vitamins, folic acid, vitamin C, magnesium, and chromium.

NOTE: For a list of recommended foods to help you manage your diet while you are on a sugar detox, turn to page 30. You'll also find a shopping list of all the ingredients that are used in the recipes and meal plans in this book on page 252.

STEP 6. Get Rid of Tempting, Sugary Foods in Your Kitchen

Some of us are prone to an external food sensitivity, which means that you get cravings when you see or smell food whether you are hungry or not. You can find out whether you have an external food sensitivity by doing the YFAS in step 3, on page 241, or by just doing a web search for an image of a milk shake, a soda, an apple pie, or whatever it is that you often crave. Sit with the image of that food for a moment. Do you notice your salivary glands moistening? Are you feeling an urge to reach through the screen and start slurping that milk shake? Perhaps your mind is distracted and you can't think of anything else *but* the milk shake. You may even be compelled to run out and buy one. If you notice these physical effects and urges, then your brain is no doubt firing off some endorphins, and you likely have an external food sensitivity.

If this is the case, then I would suggest cleaning out your kitchen to get rid of any tempting, sugary food. A recent report in *Health Education and Behavior* found that foods that are visible on kitchen countertops, particularly cereals and sodas, can predict the weight of women—and those results probably apply to men and children, too, even though the study was conducted solely with women. The study found that women whose breakfast cereals were in plain view on their kitchen counters weighed 20 pounds more than their neighbors who didn't have cereals out, and the same was true of soft drinks: women who had these items in full view in their kitchen outweighed their neighbors who did not have soft drinks on their kitchen counters by 24–26 pounds or more. Those who had a fruit bowl, however, weighed about 13 pounds less than those who didn't have a fruit bowl. The moral of this story? Get rid of that junk on your countertops and go out and get a fruit bowl!

And while you're at it, take a look at salsas, salad dressings, juice, candy, pastries, fruit and grain bars, rice cakes, syrups, processed flours, cereals, and instant oatmeal. All of these items have some sugar in them. Try to remove as many temptations as possible to set yourself up for success. If you live with roommates, friends, or family who are not particularly supportive of your dietary needs, consider a compromise. Out of sight is out of mind: Hide tempting foodstuffs behind cartons in the fridge or behind boxes and cans on pantry shelves. This may seem like a dramatic approach, but you'll be surprised how strong cravings can be. As a kid in a relatively sugar-free home, I would feel tempted every time I opened a kitchen cabinet. There before me I'd see a box of powdered hot cocoa mix staring right back at me. More often than not, I would just tear open a packet and down it without even "watering" it down . . . *Sheesh!*

Finally, I'm going to sound like a nagging mother and urge you to keep your kitchen clean and organized to the best of your ability. Why? Cluttered, chaotic kitchens turn out to be caloric booby traps. Another study reveals that when women under stressful situations were asked to wait in a messy kitchen for another person, they ended up eating twice as many cookies compared to women in the same kitchen when it was organized and quiet. In total they ate 53 more calories from cookies in 10 minutes. The lesson here is get rid of your triggers, switch out poor snacks with healthy ones, and keep that kitchen cleaned, organized, and free of sugary temptations!

STEP 7. To Stop Sugar Cravings, You Need to Quit Eating Sugar—Not Cut Back

It's far easier to follow a program when restrictions are black and white. One little bit of sugar can actually set you off on a downward spiral, so it's best to remove added sugars completely from your diet. There are ways to do this gradually. If you want to take that route, keep in mind that abstaining is *not* about "going on a diet." An alcoholic doesn't go to a support group to "go on a diet" from alcohol. Abstinence is about removing a harmful substance altogether (in this case, sugar) so that it will no longer hijack your brain chemistry. When you stop eating sugar, you will *gain* more energy, a clearer focus, and a healthier life. It will also teach you how to reprogram your taste buds and enjoy highly nutritious foods, ones that your body and mind truly need! A sugar detox plan is truly a *lifestyle* plan that will help you get closer to the source of your sugar cravings and open up new avenues for a healthier you.

There are many programs that suggest varying lengths of time for reducing or removing sugar from your diet. Behavioral research, however, shows that the length of time to correct a bad habit varies dramatically from person to person. For most of us it will take time, perhaps several weeks, months, or even years, and you may need to go back to bat several times before hitting a home run. But once you hit that home run, it will be all the sweeter—and without all the sugar!

There are several ways to quit eating sugar. **Here are two approaches:**

APPROACH 1: GRADUAL RELEASE

Remove all sodas, sugary beverages, and artificially sweetened drinks from your diet.
Most of us obtain unnecessary sugars from drinks such as soda, fruit juices, sports drinks, sweetened waters, energy drinks, sweetened teas and coffees, and even fresh-pressed juices and smoothies. Begin replacing these drinks with unsweetened beverages, including filtered tap water, sparkling water, unsweetened herbal teas, single servings of unsweetened black or green teas and coffee, or water flavored with whole fruits and herbs (see page 41 for recipes). Keep caffeinated beverages to 1 serving (6 ounces) and alcoholic beverages to 1 serving (5 ounces). Once all your cravings subside for sweetened beverages, or when you feel confident that you've built up a healthy habit of drinking unsweetened beverages, move on to the second step.

Remove other free sugars from the food you eat.
Once you've removed sugar from beverages, it's time to begin removing sugars from the rest of your diet. These items include desserts; candies; canned fruits; processed meats; dairy products, such as flavored or sweetened yogurts, processed cheese, frozen yogurt, flavored milk, and sweetened creams; frozen and prepared dinners, soups, sauces, salsas, and salad dressing; sweetened breads; sweetened granolas; crackers and chips; and alcohol. Place a particular emphasis on your breakfasts, making sure that no unwanted sugars creep in to your first meal of the day, which will only set you up for an insulin spike and subsequent cravings.

Replace refined carbohydrates with whole grains.

Once you feel as if you have sufficiently accomplished stages 1 and 2, you can move on to replacing refined carbs, such as most flours, oatmeal, white rice, breads, pizza dough, pastas, crackers, with healthier, whole(r) grain and protein options like quinoa, pearl barley, beans, and lentils.

If at any point you slip up, simply repeat the stage you're on or go back to the stage before. Remember: You're transitioning to a healthier lifestyle, and everything you do is progress, even when you slip, because you're learning how to return to a healthier foundation.

APPROACH 2: FULL RELEASE

Concentrate on eating real food (and only minimally processed food on occasion).
When I first started my sugar cleanse, I decided to quit cold turkey and removed all free sugars, processed starches, and even sugary fruits and vegetables from my diet for at least 30 days. I wanted to know what liberation from sugar would

feel like, and I was psychologically and physically prepared for the challenge. Removing everything at once can be difficult for some to maintain, but I would suggest giving the full release method a try for a specific period of time—say 10 days, 30 days, or 2 months. This will give you a sense of what life without sugar is like. Most people feel and see the results—from clearer skin to more balanced energy to weight loss— almost instantly, and all of these can be motivating factors to continue. If you ever feel that a full release from sugar is too difficult to maintain and you find yourself slipping up, analyze your food journal to learn more about your pitfalls, and then create your own personalized gradual release plan.

Though removing all added sugars and processed foods from your diet may seem extreme, it is a valid approach for some people. Author Michael Moss, in his book *Salt, Sugar, Fat*, retells a story about one of the foremost experts in addictive behavior, Nora Volkow, a research psychiatrist and scientist who directs the National Institute on Drug Abuse. Volkow pioneered the use of brain imaging to discover parallels between food and narcotics, giving more validity to food addiction. She found that processed sugar in certain individuals—including you, perhaps—can produce compulsive patterns of intake. In these situations, she recommends staying away from sugar completely. As you go through the Yale Food Addiction Survey (YFAS) on page 243, learn more about your sugar cravings, and consult with your nutritionist or health practitioner, you'll be able to determine which approach is best for you. And if you'd like to do a guided cleanse, then I encourage you to visit SugarDetox.me to sign up for one of our programs so that we can help you on your path.

STEP 8. Plan Your Meals in Advance and Make Sure You Have a Plan B for Special Occasions

It's far easier to follow a sugar detox plan when you have a list of ingredients and recipes that you can use that simplifies the steps in order to remove as many barriers as possible, which is what this book is all about. This helps you transition from eating unhealthy sugars, whether it happens gradually or as soon as you finish reading this book.

Chapter 5 (page 56) is the heart of this book, where you'll find around 80 sugar-free recipes to make planning meals over the course of a whole month easy, delicious, and inexpensive. You'll find yourself turning to these recipes again and again. I do!

Making contingency plans for special occasions is vital, whether it's a last-minute trip or a special event like a birthday or wedding, because it's all too easy to get caught off guard. When I did my initial sugar detox, it happened to coincide with Independence Day, one of two days in the year that my family gets together. I gave my aunt, who was responsible for making most of the food, a heads up that I was removing added sugar from my diet. She was wholly supportive because her husband, my uncle, had already transitioned to becoming a vegan for health reasons, and she was used to being flexible about meals.

When I arrived, the salad had already been prepared, but the dressing was off to the side; clams were being steamed; and there were plenty of veggies to eat. On that occasion, my aunt was responsive to my needs, but obviously this can't always be the case for every event, where you may not know whom the organizer is or what will be on the menu. This can be challenging if you're avoiding sugary foods, so I would suggest that you eat a proper meal beforehand, if you can, to reduce your hunger; bring snacks, like nuts, as a contingency plan; and eat lightly at the event if the food seems suspect. If you prefer not to do that, then just relax and enjoy the meal—regardless of whether it's laced with sugar or not—and don't dwell on it! The next meal will give you an opportunity to jump back on track again, because now you have a plan to rely on.

STEP 9. Find Support

We're social creatures by nature, and we often find ourselves eating in the company of others—whether at work on a lunch break, at home with family, or out on a dinner date. When I decided that I would do a sugar cleanse, it was natural for me to tell all of my friends. I emailed everyone in advance, letting them know what I was doing and why. Instead of deciding to isolate myself from the crowd, I did the opposite. I knew I would be cooking nearly every day, so I told my friends that I would like to cook for them when time would allow. Since so many of my peers in New York City go out to eat or rely on food delivery services, a home-cooked meal is viewed as something special. As I started to invite friends over for dinner—cooking for a few people about once a week—I was astonished by how inspired and interested they were in doing a detox with me. Simply opening my home and inviting conversation turned into something positive for others. This type of support within your network is indispensable to achieving success. Let your family and friends know about what you're doing, and see if they'll join you on your journey, even if it's just for one meal. If your family and friends are less than supportive, then go outside of your community, perhaps with others who are reading this book or who have joined the online community, so that you can commune with like-minded people. If you really feel as if you need professional help beyond your support group, I would encourage you to seek that help.

STEP 10. Help Yourself by Helping Others

Helping people in general is a good thing, so good that the initial euphoria you get from knowing you helped someone releases a little bit of dopamine—the happy hormone. Once you start to form bonds with other people and establish friendships, your body also begins to release serotonin and oxytocin, which allow you to feel more deeply attached to others. This is a truly natural way to feel good. And if you have looked into or actually been part of a recovery program, the last step is always helping others to overcome the same problem.

Chances are if you're achieving some success in your life, or even going through a particularly rough patch, the very act of opening up will allow both you and others to feel better. Last year, I began opening up my home for an hour of group meditation every month. We come together to sit in silence and then spend the last 45 minutes of the hour listening to one another and talking about what's on our minds. It's a safe space where people can come together to commune, without being judged. Most of us find that our challenges are not unique and that the people we know are often confronted by the same issues and go through the same emotions that we happen to be experiencing. By sharing your journey, your own actions will inspire others (and you'll be inspired by theirs), which is a powerful positive feedback loop that will naturally keep you satisfied—without the sugar!

CHAPTER 3

PREPPING YOUR **DETOX** KITCHEN & PANTRY

There's quite a bit you need to know about your own life as well as how sugar can affect your health before you get to healthy food choices. Once you're armed with that, however, you can begin to lay the groundwork for cooking in the kitchen. In this chapter you'll find suggestions for the basics—from which appliances, tools, and ingredients to buy, including pantry staples, spices, herbs, and more, to how to organize your kitchen.

25 KITCHEN APPLIANCES AND TOOLS

The kitchen appliances and tools listed below are by no means must-haves, and there's no need to buy the fanciest brands. I've cooked some delicious recipes with only a pocketknife and a single pot over an open flame, but the following will definitely make your time in the kitchen more efficient and, most important, more enjoyable.

1. BAKING DISHES (GLASS)

Glass baking dishes are durable and perfect for cooking roasts, fish, and veggies. The 2-, 3-, and 5-quart sizes are particularly handy.

2. BAKING SHEETS

Baking sheets with nonstick surfaces are great, but if you have old baking sheets, you can always use parchment paper to prevent sticking.

3. BENCH SCRAPER

I find a bench scraper useful for scooping up chopped fruits and veggies and cleaning off the cutting board. I have one with a straight edge on one side (for scooping and cleaning) and a curved edge on the other (for scraping bowls).

4. BLENDER OR FOOD PROCESSOR

A blender is the one appliance I would splurge on, because I've found that cheaply made ones can break easily, and you'll soon find yourself shopping for another one. Do yourself a favor and buy a good-quality blender and/or food processor to chop vegetables and make soups, salsas, and sauces.

5. BOWLS (VARIOUS SIZES)

Make sure you have a nice selection of bowls of all sizes for mixing and serving. I

even like to have ramekins or custard cups handy, which are perfect for singling out eggs for poaching.

6. BREAD KNIFE

The serrated edges on a bread knife are perfect for cutting rye or sourdough loaves while minimizing the crumbs. I also find that they are particularly good for cutting tomatoes.

7. CAN OPENER

Some of the recipes in this book call for canned products, so it's convenient to have a good can opener on hand.

8. CLAY POT

I particularly love cooking in clay pots because they help meats, stews, and soups retain so much moisture and flavor. I use a clay pot for the oven for roasting a whole chicken and another for the stovetop for stews, which is also safe for oven use.

9. CHEF'S KNIFE

A good chef's knife is worth its weight in gold. This is the knife that you will be using the majority of the time, so it's important to get a good one and keep it sharp.

10. COLANDER OR SALAD SPINNER

Certain greens, like lettuce and spinach, can retain a lot of water after washing and are a pain to dry, so I suggest getting a good salad spinner, which can double as a colander.

11. PRESSURE COOKER

A pressure cooker is basically an airtight pot with a sealable lid used to heat food evenly and cook it quickly. You can even use it for canning. If you are often short on time, I would highly recommend investing in a pressure cooker because it can cut your cooking time in half! A pressure cooker is particularly useful for making broths, grains, meats, soups, and stews. Please note that cooking times will vary depending on the model.

12. GRATERS

It's great to have a number of graters in your arsenal, for example, a box grater for grating veggies, like cauliflower and carrots; a microplane zester for citrus zesting; and a mandoline for slicing thin pieces of beets, carrots, turnips, potatoes, and other root vegetables.

13. IMMERSION BLENDER

Immersion blenders are not absolutely necessary, particularly if you already have a blender or food processor, but I find them easier to use, particularly when cooking hot soups that you want to go from chunky to creamy. It's a lot easier to use an immersion blender on the stovetop or counter than it is to transport a heavy pot to a blender or food processor and transfer the hot contents to the machine.

14. MEASURING CUPS AND SPOONS

Some cooks forgo measuring cups and spoons and just eyeball amounts. This is fine if you are an experienced cook or if you feel confident in the kitchen, but if you don't, pick up some measuring cups and spoons.

15. PARCHMENT BAKING PAPER

Parchment paper is used as a nonstick liner for baking dishes and baking sheets. I particularly love the paper because it reduces cleanup time, especially when you're using olive oil on your ingredients. I use it often when roasting mushrooms, squash, and other veggies.

16. PEELER

I prefer to keep the skin on most of my fruits and veggies, but occasionally I prefer the skin off, for example, when I'm making a creamy soup. That's when a good peeler comes in handy.

17. PLATES (SMALL, LARGE)

Plates seem to be a no-brainer, but I've included them here for a reason: Begin training yourself to eat main courses—particularly ones where vegetables are the centerpiece—on large plates, and if you decide to eat desserts once your cleanse is done, begin eating them on small plates to help manage portions.

18. SAUCEPANS

Saucepans of various sizes are great to have on hand, but I've found that a medium-size saucepan is the most useful for making small amounts of soups, sauces, and reheating leftovers.

19. SIEVE

Get yourself a stainles-steel fine-mesh strainer or sieve. I particularly like colanders with a handle and grips, so you can strain what you have over another pot. This utensil is critical when making broths and teas and when sifting through grains to clean them before cooking.

20. SKILLET

I have two skillets: a medium to large nonstick skillet for the stovetop and another skillet that is oven safe. The latter is a particularly good choice when you want to sear meat on the stovetop and then finish it off in the oven.

21. SLOTTED SPOON

I love poaching eggs and find that a slotted spoon is the easiest way to retrieve them from a hot water bath.

22. SPATULA (METAL)

I use many kinds of spatulas, including a fish spatula, a flexible, slotted tool that is often used for more delicate food items, but a simple metal spatula is the way to go for most food items.

23. SPATULA (RUBBER, VARIOUS SIZES)

A rubber spatula is handy for scooping mixtures out of your food processor or blender.

24. SPIRALIZER

A spiralizer is not necessary, but once you have one, you'll notice a difference in your enjoyment of veggies and presentation of dishes.

A spiralizer comes with multiple blades that allow you to create many different vegetable shapes from "noodles" to short curls.

25. ALUMINUM FOIL

Aluminum foil is necessary, particularly if you need to keep steam in when baking a dish. It can also be used instead of parchment paper to keep food from sticking to your baking sheets. I prefer to buy heavy-duty foil so that I can reuse it.

PREPARING YOUR KITCHEN

Be sure to keep your kitchen well organized so that you'll know where everything is. You'll want to make sure that your appliances, tools, and other items are easy to access, particularly if you use them again and again. You'll be surprised how little things make a big difference. For instance, I hang my measuring cups on a ring, but since I use the ½ cup and 1 cup measurements most often, they hang off the ring so that I can grab them more easily. Second, since I'm a big tea drinker—even in the summer months—my kettle is always on the stovetop, ready to go as soon as I wake up in the morning. Third, I love having my spices and herbs within arm's reach. Last, I love having access to fresh herbs that I can clip as I cook. Buying cut herbs from the store can add up, and if you don't use all of them, the rest goes into the compost bin. For the same price, you can buy potted herbs and snip off whatever you need when you need it. I typically have basil, thyme, sage, oregano, and rosemary growing indoors. Organizing your kitchen sensibly will ultimately save you time and make cooking far more enjoyable.

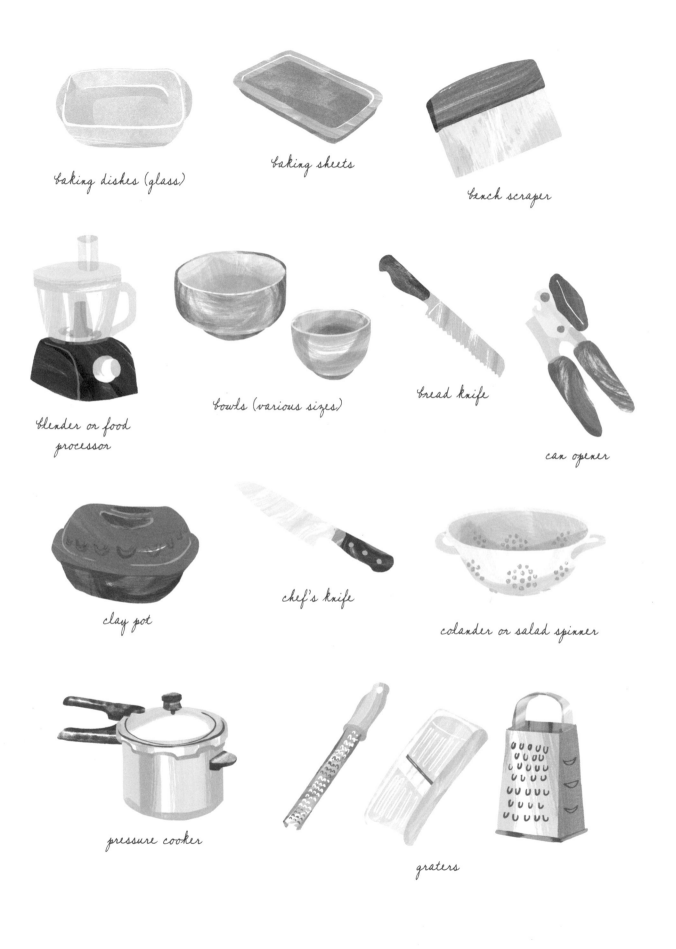

baking dishes (glass)

baking sheets

bench scraper

blender or food processor

bowls (various sizes)

bread knife

can opener

clay pot

chef's knife

colander or salad spinner

pressure cooker

graters

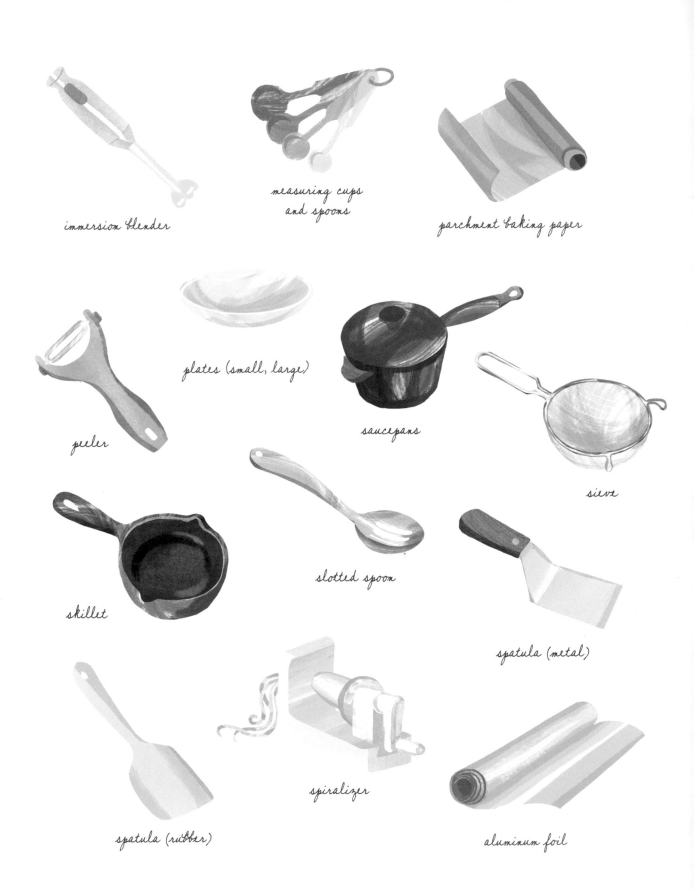

immersion blender

measuring cups
and spoons

parchment baking paper

peeler

plates (small, large)

saucepans

sieve

skillet

slotted spoon

spatula (metal)

spatula (rubber)

spiralizer

aluminum foil

CHOOSING MEAT

You'll notice that the majority of recipes in this book are veggie-centric. I'm a big proponent of reducing your meat intake to around 5 percent of your diet or less and practice "meat only on Mondays" instead of "meatless Mondays." I suggest limiting your intake of red meat to two servings per month. If you eat meat, try not to overcook it because this releases carcinogenic, or cancer-causing, compounds. Also consider alternatives to red meat, like wild meat (e.g., venison) and, of course, chicken. Try to opt for pastured, certified organic meats that were treated humanely, as animals fed on corn and grain meals will not be as nutritious. Also note that when buying red meat, the USDA recently revoked the "grass-fed" label, so it's now rendered virtually meaningless. However, if you're lucky to know your farmer or your local butcher, ask them whether their animals were truly grass-fed or not.

CHOOSING WHOLE GRAINS

True whole grains contain all ingredients within a kernel, which means the starchy endosperm, the bran (the outer skin of the kernel), and the germ (the embryo on the inside that has the ability to sprout a new plant). The bran and the germ contain all the fiber, some protein, healthy fats, and phytochemicals. The process of refining starches removes the germ and the bran and therefore strips the grain of its nutrients, leaving only the sugars. You'll want to eat as much of the intact grain as possible. The key here is intact grain, because our breads and packaged products can say "whole grain" without being truly whole. I know, it's frustrating and confusing. Here is a surefire way to figure out whether something is whole grain—or at least more whole. Flip to the back of the ingredients list. They are listed in order by weight, so breads, for example, should have ingredients like whole kernel rye, cracked wheat, bran, and rolled oats. However, packaged bread—the ones we typically see at our supermarket—will likely only have ingredients like unbleached enriched flour (wheat flour, malted barley flour, niacin, reduced iron, thiamin mononitrate, riboflavin, folic acid), water, honey, sugar, wheat gluten. Steer clear of those breads, pastas, and other prepared starches!

CHOOSING OILS

When using oils, I like to stick to organic coconut oil and cold-pressed olive oil and flaxseed oil. I will occasionally use sesame oil, but not in excess. Stay away from canola, corn, cottonseed, safflower, and soy oils, as these oils are highly processed and the majority of them are high in omega-6 fatty acids. Omega-6 fatty acids are important to the body in small doses, but in general, we have too much of them in our body, due to a high intake of processed foods. A surfeit of omega-6 can lead to metabolic disorders, including insulin resistance, so we'll want to keep them in check.

CORE INGREDIENTS

Even though I encourage people to have a diverse diet, the purpose of this book is to supply you with all the ingredients and recipes you'll need to help you achieve your sugar detox goals. To that end, core ingredient focus on about 100 items that you'll use over and over again. If you have specific allergies and need to replace certain ingredients, want to experiment with different fruits and vegetables, or don't like the taste of a particular ingredient, then by all means feel free to use an alternative ingredient that works for you; there's a more complete, though not exhaustive list, in Appendix D on page 252 that you can use as a guide. The 100 items in the core list are there to help reduce the barrier of temptation as much as possible when you're grocery shopping. One way to do that is by selecting a list of ingredients, creating a shopping list, and sticking to it!

Apple, green	Endive	Onion, red	Sole
Artichokes	Garlic	Onion, shallot	Spinach
Asparagus	Ghee	Onion, yellow	Squash, acorn
Avocado	Ginger	Parsnips	Squash, butternut
Bacon	Halibut	Peas	Squash, kabocha
Banana	Kale, curly	Pepper, green bell	Squash, spaghetti
Barley, pearl	Kale, lacinato	Pepper, jalapeño	Stock/broth
Beans, mung	Kefir	Pepper, red bell	Tahini paste
Beets	Lemon	Pine nuts	Tomato, cherry
Bok choy	Lime	Pomegranate	Tomato, heirloom
Bread, rye	Microgreens	Quinoa	Tomato, plum
Bread, sourdough	Mushrooms, button	Potato, regular	Tomato, sun-dried
Broccoli	Mushrooms, cremini	Potato, sweet	Turnips
Brussels sprouts	Mushrooms, enoki	Pork, ham	Vinegar (apple cider,
Cabbage, green	Mushrooms, oyster	Pork, kielbasa	balsamic, distilled,
Cabbage, red	Mushrooms,	Pork, minced	red, rice, sherry,
Carrots	portobello	Radish, watermelon	white wine)
Cauliflower	Mustard	Radish, regular	Zucchini, green
Celery	Mustard greens	Salmon	Zucchini, yellow
Chicken	Nuts, almonds	Sauce, tamari	
Chiles	Nuts, walnuts	Sauerkraut	
Chorizo	Oil, extra virgin olive	Seaweed, wakame	
Coconut milk	Oil, sesame	Seaweed snacks	
Coconut oil	Onion, green	Seeds, sesame	
Cucumber	(scallions)	Seeds, sunflower	
Eggs	Onion, leek	Shrimp	

BASIC INGREDIENTS TO HAVE ON HAND

Once you've organized your kitchen, you'll want to make sure you always have some basic pantry staples on hand. Try to buy in bulk where you can—it'll save you money in the long run and also reduce your grocery bills when you go out to buy fresh items.

OILS AND VINEGARS

Coconut oil

Extra virgin olive oil

Flaxseed oil

Ghee

Sesame oil

Vinegar (apple cider, balsamic, distilled, rice, sherry, white wine)

FRUITS, VEGGIES, AND ROOTS

Garlic

Ginger

Lemon

Lime

Onion, red

Onion, yellow

Shallots

SPICES

Cayenne

Cinnamon

Cumin

Curry

Ginger

Nutmeg

Pepper

Red pepper flakes

Saffron

Sea Salt

Turmeric

Vanilla extract

FLOURS, ETC.

Almond flour

Carob powder

Coconut flour

NUTS AND SEEDS

Almonds

Pine nuts

Sesame seeds

Sunflower seeds

Walnuts

PULSES AND GRAINS

Barley, pearl

Beans

Lentils

Quinoa

STOCKS AND BROTHS

Chicken broth

Mushroom broth

Vegetable broth

SAUCES AND SPREADS

Almond butter

Tahini paste

Tamari sauce

What's wonderful about the basic ingredients in these lists is that if they are stored properly, they'll keep for some time. Even fresh items, like lemons and limes, can be kept for weeks in the crisper—and when they get a little soft, they are still perfectly fine for juicing, baking, and zesting, which is what we'll be using them for in any case.

FOR THE PANTRY

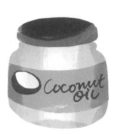

coconut oil

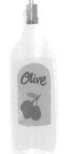

extra virgin
olive oil

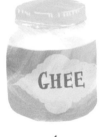

ghee

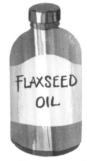

flaxseed oil

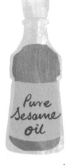

sesame oil

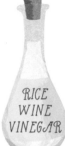

rice vinegar

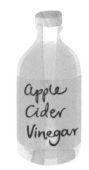

apple cider vinegar

balsamic vinegar

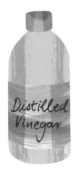

distilled vinegar

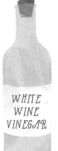

red wine vinegar

white wine vinegar

sherry vinegar

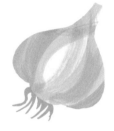

garlic

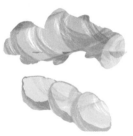

ginger

lemon

lime

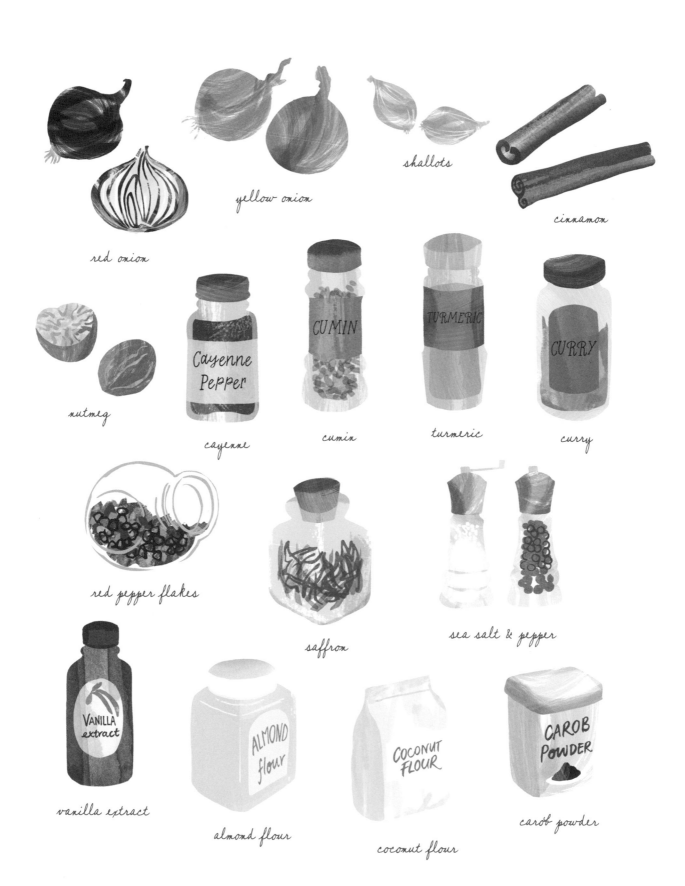

red onion

yellow onion

shallots

cinnamon

nutmeg

Cayenne Pepper

cayenne

CUMIN

cumin

TURMERIC

turmeric

CURRY

curry

red pepper flakes

saffron

sea salt & pepper

VANILLA extract

vanilla extract

ALMOND flour

almond flour

COCONUT FLOUR

coconut flour

CAROB POWDER

carob powder

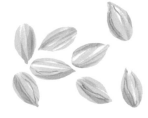

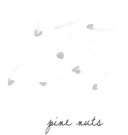

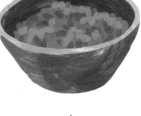

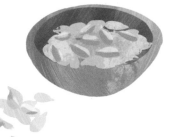

almonds

pine nuts

sesame seeds

sunflower seeds

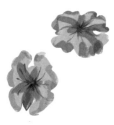

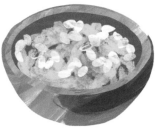

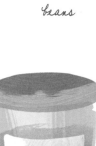

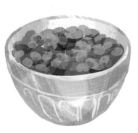

walnuts

barley

beans

lentils

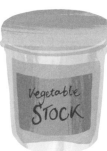

quinoa

chicken broth

mushroom broth

vegetable broth

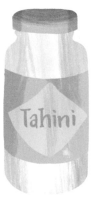

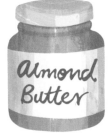

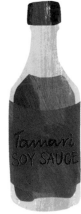

tahini paste

almond butter

tamari sauce

GROWING HERBS

If you have an outdoor growing space, fire escape, balcony, or direct light in your home, I encourage growing some of your favorite herbs. If you've never grown a plant before, then start small—maybe two or three of your favorite herbs, like basil, rosemary, and mint. Start growing them in separate containers, because they'll prefer slightly different watering regimes, and if one is affected by bugs, then it'll less likely infect another plant if it is separate from the start. Herbs require quite a bit of sun, so arrange them in a south-facing window where they'll get direct light. Growing herbs indoors is superior to buying fresh herbs: You'll save money, you can use them when you need them, and your herbs will be superfresh, which means there's no need to freeze or compost them.

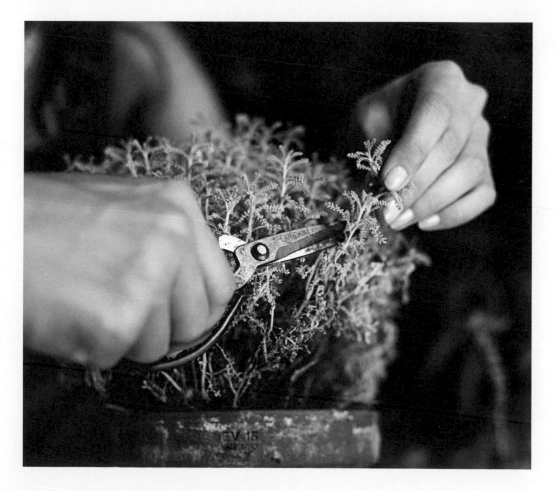

HERBS AND BEST USES

Basil—pestos, tomato salad, salad dressing, soups, poultry, and iced and hot drinks

Bay—bouquet garni, soups, stews, stocks, marinades, pickles, fish, tomato sauce, beans, lentils, lamb

Chives—yogurts, fish, potatoes, zucchini, root vegetables, eggs

Cilantro—soups, salad dressings, sauces, tacos, fish, guacamole

Dill—fish, pickling, salad dressings, cabbage, cauliflower, cucumber, savory yogurts, salads

Lemongrass—hot drinks, salad dressing, soup, stews, chicken, pork, fish, shellfish

Mint—tea, carrots, peas, fruit salad, drinks, lamb, pork, chicken, hot and cold drinks

Oregano—roasted vegetables, tomato sauce, stews, soups, vinegars

Parsley—bouquet garni, salads, salad dressings, fish, lentils, roasted veggies

Rosemary—marinades, chicken, lamb, olive oil, cold drinks, cabbage, eggplant, lentils, mushrooms, squash

Thyme—bouquet garni, stews, soups, chicken, sauces, salad dressings, cabbage, potatoes, mushrooms

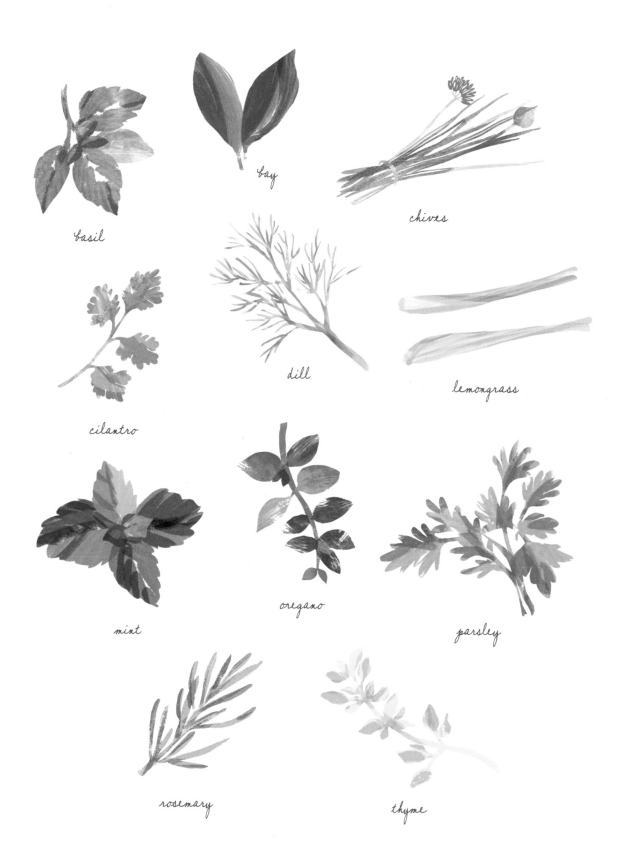

basil

bay

chives

cilantro

dill

lemongrass

mint

oregano

parsley

rosemary

thyme

EIGHT EASY TECHNIQUES TO CURB SUGAR TOOTH

1. Drink water before your meals. Oftentimes when we think we're hungry, it's really our body telling us we're dehydrated.

2. Be sure to eliminate sugar at breakfast. You'll have more even energy throughout the day and will eventually reduce cravings more naturally.

3. Limit yourself to around two servings of sweeter whole fruits throughout the day, though it's okay to eat more if you're craving free sugars. Remember: whole fruit with the fiber is far better than free sugars!

4. Slow down when you eat. Though we're often compelled to eat quickly, be mindful and put your fork down from time to time. Additionally, if you're eating courses or going up for seconds, allow around 20 minutes before you dive in. It can take our brain a while to catch up and acknowledge that we're not hungry.

5. Snack between meals if you're really hungry. This is okay to do; it just depends on what you're snacking on! Try to munch on something that is no more than 100 calories and does not contain free sugar, like a handful of raw nuts, a spoonful of nut butter, olives, or even a whole fruit.

6. If you're eating something sweet, exercise portion control. Place it on a smaller dish and eat it with a smaller spoon or fork. We tend to eat less when we have a smaller plate and smaller utensils.

7. Don't eat before bedtime. If you have an empty stomach before the evening hours, your body will more likely burn fat. Try to eat 2–3 hours before bedtime.

8. Read your labels! Though nutrition labels can be confusing, by arming ourselves with the knowledge of how to read them, we'll become more empowered eaters.

CHAPTER 4

BASIC RECIPES: SNACKS, DRINKS, DRESSINGS & SAUCES

When we think of eating healthfully, we often have images of mealtime: breakfast, lunch, and dinner. We less often consider what's in between or on the side: the drinks, the dressings, the snacks, and the sauces. A big salad paired with a creamy Thousand Island dressing, a glass of apple juice, and a handful of crackers will give you more added sugar than you require in a given day, compliments of the dressing, the drink, and the snack.

But snacking is not inherently bad. Before sitting down for dinner became so "American"—a tradition that largely started in the 1880s and was fortified at the turn of the twentieth century—snacking was quite common. But the concept of spoiling your appetite between meals has really stuck in our culture, giving snacking a bad rap. Where snacking can become a slippery slope is threefold: what we're snacking on, how much we're snacking, and how mindless the activity has become, meaning we often snack on autopilot. Snacks like cookies, chips, candies, and energy bars have become ubiquitous in vending machines, in corner delis, on trains and subways, in hospitals, at workplaces, and in supermarkets. Snack foods today are typically energy dense and, if processed, contain very little nutritional value.

Sauces, spreads, and dressings also used to be *au natural*, and it wasn't until recently—over the last 30–40 years or so—that we started to see an uptick of sugar in everything from tomato sauces to our condiments. I've learned to stick to a handful of healthy snacks, and where I can, I make my own dressings, sauces, and drinks. What's even better is that it's quick, easy, and affordable to do.

SNACKS

Though our supermarket shelves are filled with unhealthy snacks, there are quite a few that I particularly love. Here are some of my go-to snacks:

- Almond nut butter or sunflower butter
- Artichokes in olive oil
- Celery sticks (paired with nut butter)
- Olives
- Unsalted and salted nuts (e.g., almonds, pistachios)
- Seaweed snacks
- Whole fruit

THREE-INGREDIENT "ICE CREAM"

If you miss the cool, smooth texture of ice cream while you're on a sugar cleanse, try this delicious substitute. It's easy and there are only three ingredients!

1 whole banana, sliced and frozen

½ cup nut milk

2 tablespoons raw almond butter

Put all the ingredients in a blender and puree them until they're smooth. If you'd like to add a little spice, sprinkle in some cinnamon.

DRINKS

If you want to have something a bit more exciting than tap water, sparkling water, or unsweetened teas and coffee, then try some of these recipes.

APPLE, MINT, AND STRAWBERRY TEA

This recipe was inspired by the whole fruit teas that are concocted at my local café. Although you can serve it hot or cold, I particularly love it hot, even in warm weather, because the heat from the water releases the naturally sweet flavor from the fruit. As your taste buds start to reacclimate, you'll find that the flavors of whole fruit are perfectly satisfying.

5 MINUTES   **2** SERVINGS   VEGAN

INGREDIENTS

⅓ cup green apple, diced

¼ cup strawberries, diced

2-3 sprigs mint leaves

2¼ cups boiling water

DIRECTIONS

Place the apple, strawberries, and mint in a teapot. Add the water and let steep for 2 minutes. Enjoy.

LEMONGRASS, BASIL, AND PINEAPPLE TEA

I used to eat so much pineapple during the summer months that my tongue would sting, due to the enzyme bromelain, which is used as both a meat tenderizer and an anti-inflammatory. As a hot tea, however, the pineapple is sipped, rather than scarfed down as a whole fruit, and the lemongrass and basil provide some herbaceous notes to balance out pineapple's citrusy sweetness.

5 MINUTES   **2** SERVINGS   VEGAN

INGREDIENTS

⅓ cup pineapple, diced

1 3-inch lemongrass stem

2-3 sprigs of basil (I prefer lemon or cinnamon basil)

2¼ cups boiling water

DIRECTIONS

Place the pineapple, lemongrass, and basil in a teapot. Add the water and let the mixture steep for 2 minutes. Enjoy.

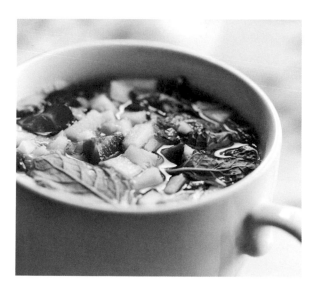

CUCUMBER-LEMON WATER

Popular in spas, cucumber-lemon water is both hydrating and refreshing. I usually serve it in the summer and early autumn for the monthly meditations I have in my home. When I ask whether a person would like regular water, sparkling water, or chilled water infused with cucumber and lemon, they most often choose the latter. It's so simple, yet so refreshing!

5 MINUTES   **4** SERVINGS   VEGAN

INGREDIENTS

1 cup sliced cucumber

1 lemon, washed and sliced

DIRECTIONS

Add the cucumber and lemon to a large flask. Fill with cold water and chill in the refrigerator. This will keep for 2–3 days before you have to compost the fruits.

WATERMELON-MINT WATER

Watermelon-mint water is the epitome of summer. The watermelon is naturally sweet while the mint brings a clean, lively flavor to the water. During August and September in the Northeast, I often get watermelons at the farmers market. Farmers know their melons are ripe for picking because there is a little curly tendril that dries out close to the melon's stem. If you want to make sure the melon you're about to purchase is perfect, just tap on the melon with two fingers; if it sounds hollow, you have a good one.

5 MINUTES   **4** SERVINGS   VEGAN

INGREDIENTS

1 cup diced watermelon

2 slices of lime

2–3 sprigs of mint

DIRECTIONS

Add the watermelon, lime, and mint to a large flask. Fill the flask with cold water and chill it in the refrigerator. The watermelon-mint water will keep for 2–3 days before you have to compost the fruits.

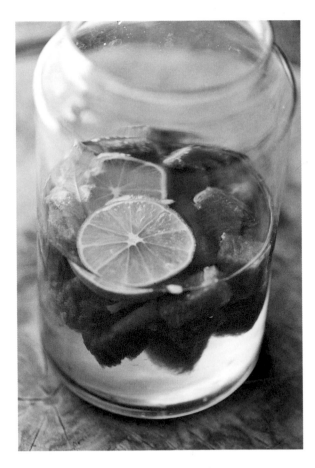

HOMEMADE ALMOND MILK

Nut milks are particularly helpful for folks like my mother, who is lactose intolerant, which simply means she can't digest the sugar in milk. If you haven't made your own almond milk yet, I encourage you to give it a try so that you can taste the difference. Typical store-bought almond milks sometimes use potentially inflammatory additives, like carrageenan, which is designed to give store-bought milk a thick, velvety "mouth feel." Freshly made almond milk, however, is light, creamy, and frothy. If you have an aversion to almonds or don't have them on hand, you can substitute them with macadamia nuts, cashews, or even coconut flakes! Adding a little cinnamon, nutmeg, vanilla extract, and even a pinch of salt will help accentuate the flavor of the nuts.

10 MINUTES   **2** SERVINGS   VEGAN

INGREDIENTS

1 cup almonds, soaked overnight

2 cups water

1 teaspoon sea salt

1 teaspoon cinnamon (optional)

1 teaspoon nutmeg (optional)

1 tablespoon vanilla extract (optional)

1. Soak the almonds overnight. Place a lid over them and keep them on your kitchen countertop or in the refrigerator.

2. Drain the soaking water. Put the almonds in a blender with 2 cups of fresh water and salt. Add optional ingredients. Blend the mixture on high for 1-2 minutes.

3. Strain the almond milk mixture through a nutbag or a cheesecloth into another wide-mouthed container. Refrigerate the milk and use it within 3 days.

FRUITS

While you're sugar detoxing, you'll want to keep your sweet fruit intake down to around two servings of whole sweet fruits per day, which is hard to do, especially in the height of summer when fruits are abundant. I specify "sweet fruit" intake because some fruits, like squash (which are considered vegetables by many anyway), have a reduced amount of fructose and are perfectly fine to nosh on liberally. However, I'd steer clear of dried fruits like dates, mangos, prunes, raisins, and peaches, which are total sugar bombs. I'd also advise only having small amounts of high-fructose fruits, like cherries, watermelons, grapes, apples, pears, and pomegranates. If you're going to eat them, try to space them out over the course of the day, as opposed to eating them all at once, or use them to naturally flavor tap water or sparkling water. See Appendix E, page 254, for a more complete list of fruits and fruit sugars.

DRESSINGS AND SAUCES

TRADITIONAL PESTO

I'm a big fan of pesto, largely because it's such a versatile condiment. Slather it on fish, a crusty slice of sourdough, or roasted root vegetables, or swirl it in soup. Want it more garlicky? Add a couple more cloves to the mix. Want a cheesy taste without the dairy? Drop in an extra ½ tablespoon of nutritional yeast. Pesto is the type of spread you can make all your own.

10 MINUTES   **4** SERVINGS   VEGAN

INGREDIENTS

1 cup basil leaves

½ cup parsley

2 garlic cloves, peeled

2 tablespoons pine nuts

¼ cup extra virgin olive oil

⅛ tablespoon nutritional yeast

Juice of 1 lemon

¼ teaspoon sea salt

⅛ teaspoon ground pepper

DIRECTIONS

Combine the basil, parsley, garlic, pine nuts, olive oil, nutritional yeast, and lemon juice in a blender and blend for 2 minutes or until smooth. Season to taste with salt and pepper.

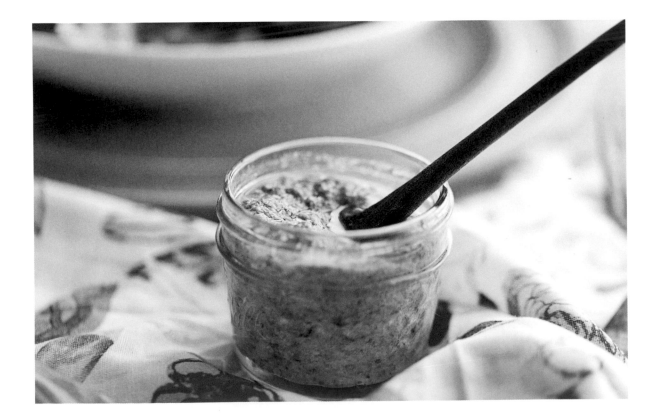

KALE PESTO

My kale pesto came about because I didn't have parsley in my garden, and then I ran out of pine nuts, so I did what any home cook would do: improvise! You can choose to soften the kale by massaging the leaves with olive oil, or, in the case of this recipe, I found blanching softens the leaves for blending and lessens the bitterness of the kale.

10 MINUTES   **4** SERVINGS   VEGAN

INGREDIENTS

1 cup kale

½ cup basil

2 garlic cloves, peeled

2 tablespoons sunflower seeds

⅓ cup extra virgin olive oil

Juice of ½ lemon

¼ teaspoon sea salt

⅛ teaspoon ground pepper

DIRECTIONS

1. Bring a medium pot of salted water to a boil.

2. Fill another bowl with ice and water.

3. Blanch the kale for 25 seconds, then remove it and place it in the ice water.

4. Dry the kale in a colander or salad spinner.

5. Combine the kale, basil, garlic, sunflower seeds, olive oil, and lemon juice in a blender and blend for 2 minutes or until smooth. Season to taste with salt and pepper.

* If you want a chunky pesto, pulse rather than blend it. If you want a creamy pesto, blend it for a couple more minutes.

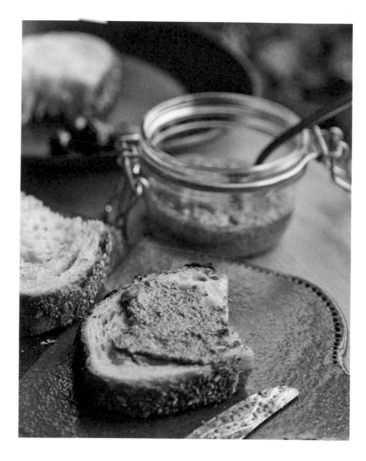

PRESTO! YOU'RE MAKING PESTO

Pesto is one of the easiest sauces to make, and it is highly versatile. Use it as a spread on breads, as a salad dressing, on roasted vegetables, in soups, and also as a dressing for meats and fish. You can use just about any green to make it, from carrot tops to spinach. And you can use just about any seed or nut, too! Just remember this equation: 1½ cups of greens + 2 garlic cloves + 2 tablespoons seeds or nuts + juice of ½ lemon + ⅓ cup extra virgin olive oil = pesto!

HOLLANDAISE SAUCE

If you've had eggs benedict, then you have had hollandaise sauce, a buttery, yellow sauce of egg yolk and, in this case, clarified butter, or ghee. Clarified butter has a higher smoke point than butter, and the milk and water have been removed from the butterfat, which means it's acceptable to anyone who is lactose intolerant.

15 MINUTES   **4** SERVINGS   VEGETARIAN

INGREDIENTS

2 egg yolks

1½ tablespoons lemon juice

⅛ teaspoon paprika

⅛ teaspoon sea salt

½ cup ghee, melted

DIRECTIONS

1. Add the egg yolks, lemon juice, paprika, and salt to a blender and blend on low for about 30 seconds. Slowly drizzle in the warm melted ghee and fully blend.

2. The sauce will emulsify and can be used immediately. If it starts to thicken, just mix in a little bit of hot water.

CHIMICHURRI SAUCE

Chimichurri sauce is an Argentinian-derived sauce chock-full of herbaceous greens, extra virgin olive oil, and red pepper flakes. Surprisingly, it didn't appear in Latin American cookbooks until 1991, according to food writer Joyce Goldstein. Chimichurri is an herby sauce that pairs well with meat, fish, and shrimp.

10 MINUTES   **4** SERVINGS   VEGAN

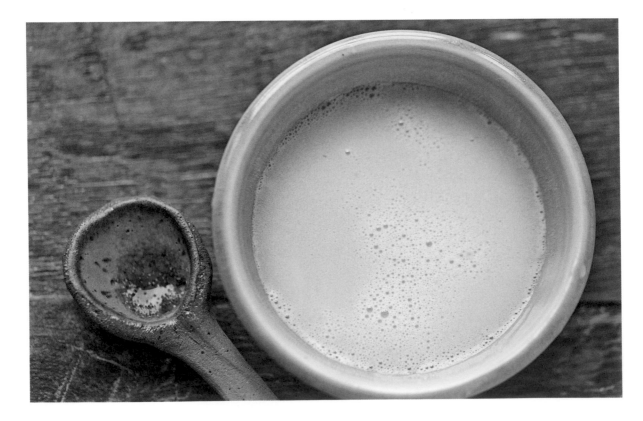

INGREDIENTS

1 cup flat leaf parsley

1 tablespoon fresh oregano

3 cloves garlic, peeled

½ cup extra virgin olive oil

1 tablespoon white wine vinegar

Juice of ¼ lemon

¼ teaspoon sea salt

⅛ teaspoon pepper, freshly ground

Red pepper flakes

DIRECTIONS

1. Add the parsley, oregano, and garlic to a blender and pulse for 30 seconds. Transfer the mixture to a bowl.

2. Stir in the olive oil, vinegar, lemon juice, salt, and pepper. Add the red pepper flakes. Taste and adjust seasonings as necessary.

TAHINI SAUCE

Tahini sauce is primarily made from tahini paste, which is made from toasted ground hulled sesame seeds and is integral to other popular spreads like hummus and baba ghanoush. Tahini imparts a nutty flavor to sauces and works particularly well with raw and roasted veggies, nori wraps, and kebabs.

10 MINUTES **4** SERVINGS VEGAN

INGREDIENTS

3 tablespoons tahini paste

Juice of 1 lemon

1 garlic clove, peeled

⅛ teaspoon cumin

⅛ teaspoon paprika

3-4 tablespoons water

¼ teaspoon sea salt

DIRECTIONS

Add the tahini, lemon juice, garlic, cumin, paprika, water, and salt to a blender and blend for about 1 minute or until the mixture is smooth.

HARISSA

Harissa is a hot chile sauce that became popular in Northern Africa, after chile peppers from Central and South America were introduced in the 15th and 16th centuries. You can add more heat to the sauce by adding more chiles or leaving in some seeds.

35 MINUTES **4** SERVINGS VEGAN

INGREDIENTS

2 red bell peppers, sliced in half, seeds removed

1 cup boiling water

4 dried chile peppers (ancho or guajillo*)

1 garlic clove

1 tablespoon lemon juice

1 teaspoon cumin

½ teaspoon smoked paprika

2 tablespoons extra virgin olive oil

½ teaspoon sea salt

* If you are using guajillo peppers, you may need to soak them a little longer

DIRECTIONS

1. Roast the bell peppers at 450°F for 25–30 minutes or until the skin begins to char. Place them in a bowl and cover with plastic wrap until the skin starts to separate from the peppers. Remove the skins.

2. While the peppers are roasting, pour the boiling water into a bowl over the dried chiles. Let the chiles soak for 20–30 minutes until they soften. Cut off the tops and remove the seeds. Put them into a blender.

3. Add the roasted bell peppers, garlic, lemon juice, cumin, and smoked paprika to the blender. Pulse the ingredients until a paste forms, Add a little olive oil and salt for taste.

DIRECTIONS

1. Place the egg yolks, lemon juice, salt, and pepper into a blender and blend on low.

2. Add the garlic cloves and blend for 15 seconds. Slowly pour in the olive oil and continue to blend until the mixture is emulsified.

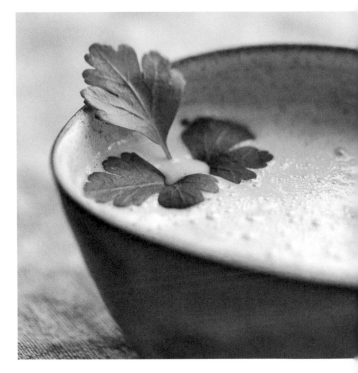

AIOLI

Aioli simply means "oil and garlic." It is particularly delicious paired with artichokes, asparagus, and portobello mushrooms or drizzled over kale salad, sweet potatoes, cauliflower, and meats.

15 MINUTES   **8** SERVINGS   VEGETARIAN

INGREDIENTS

2 medium egg yolks

2 tablespoons lemon juice

Pinch of sea salt

⅛ teaspoon white pepper

2 small garlic cloves, peeled

¾ cup extra virgin olive oil

SALSA

Sure, salsa is easy to buy, but it's also easy to make—and nothing beats freshly made salsa, particularly if you have access to in-season tomatoes. Instead of scarfing it down with chips, try pairing this salsa with some baked white fish or on chicken, a vegetable, fish ceviche, or even your eggs—baked, scrambled, or any other way.

35 MINUTES   **4** SERVINGS   VEGAN

INGREDIENTS

¾ cup diced tomato

½ tablespoon diced red onion

1 garlic clove, peeled and diced

2 tablespoons diced jalapeño pepper, no seeds

2 tablespoons diced green pepper

1 tablespoon roughly chopped cilantro

1 tablespoon diced peeled mango

Juice of 1 lime

⅛ teaspoon cumin

Pinch of sea salt

⅛ teaspoon white pepper

DIRECTIONS

Combine all the ingredients in a bowl. Mix well. Cover and refrigerate the salsa for about 30 minutes before serving.

¼ teaspoon cayenne (optional)

¼ teaspoon saffron threads (optional)

Two sprigs of dill (optional)

⅓ cup extra virgin olive oil

Juice and zest of one lemon

Sea salt, to taste

DIRECTIONS

1. Press or pound the ginger into a paste.

2. Add the parsley, cilantro, garlic, cumin, cayenne, saffron, and dill.

3. Slowly pour in the olive oil in a steady stream while blending to form an emulsion.

4. Transfer the sauce to a bowl and stir in the lemon juice and lemon zest. Season with salt, cover and place in the fridge. Let it sit for 1–2 hours for the sauce to marinate, if possible.

CHERMOULA

Like harissa, chermoula originated in North Africa. It is used to season shrimp and fish, but you can also spread it over baked eggs, sourdough bread, and vegetables.

75 MINUTES   **2** SERVINGS   VEGAN

INGREDIENTS

½ tablespoon grated ginger

3 tablespoons flat leaf parsley, finely chopped

3 tablespoons cilantro, chopped

1 garlic clove, finely chopped

1 teaspoon cumin

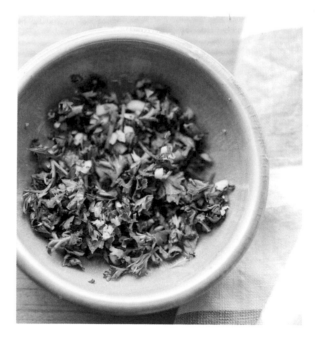

GREMOLATA

Gremolata is not quite a sauce or a spread, but I wanted to include it here since this lovely combo of parsley, garlic, and citrus notes can elevate so many dishes. Sprinkle it on top of salads, use it as a rub for meat, add it to fish and shrimp dishes, and or use it to dress up roasted roots or grilled vegetables. The possibilities for this fresh, springy, citrusy Italian-inspired condiment are endless!

10 MINUTES **2** SERVINGS VEGAN

INGREDIENTS

1 cup finely chopped parsley

Zest of 1 lemon

Juice of ½ lemon

1 garlic clove, peeled and finely chopped

Pinch of sea salt

DIRECTIONS

Put all the ingredients in a bowl and mix well. If they aren't chopped finely enough to your liking, add them to a blender and pulse for a few seconds, or place all the ingredients in the bowl of a food processor and process in short pulses until the mixture is finely chopped, but not pureed: you should still be able to make out individual flecks of citrus zest and parsley. Alternatively, you can chop the ingredients by hand.

THREE-INGREDIENT SALAD DRESSING

Salads are a go-to meal because they are quick, easy, and nutritious. You can use this recipe as a base for just about any dressing. Add watermelon or some herbs to the mix and bam—you've got yourself a whole new twist and taste!

Juice of 1 lemon

1 tablespoon extra virgin olive oil

Sprinkle of Maldon sea salt

Mix all the ingredients in a bowl until they're thoroughly incorporated. Add the dressing to your salad and enjoy!

SHALLOT–WHITE WINE VINAIGRETTE

Shallots are my onions of choice when it comes to making a dressing. They are smaller and a little harder to peel than their larger onion counterparts, but the effort is well worth it. When you're peeling shallots, try to remove as few of the outer layers as possible, because that's where the highest concentration of bioflavonoids are, particularly quercetin, which has been shown to improve gut and cardiovascular health and reduce inflammation.

15 MINUTES **4** SERVINGS VEGAN

INGREDIENTS

1 medium shallot, finely minced

2 tablespoons white wine vinegar

1 tablespoon finely chopped flat leaf parsley

¼ cup extra virgin olive oil

¼ teaspoon sea salt

DIRECTIONS

1. Put the shallot, vinegar, and parsley in a bowl. Slowly stir in the olive oil until the mixture is well integrated.

2. Add a sprinkling of salt.

BASIL-WALNUT SOAK

Instead of adding whole nuts, like walnuts or pecans, to your salad (I always have trouble spearing them with my fork), try blending them with some fresh herbs and some extra virgin olive oil or flaxseed oil. You'll get just as much nutty flavor from the dressing—and it'll be better incorporated throughout the salad.

15 MINUTES   **4** SERVINGS   VEGAN

INGREDIENTS

½ cup extra virgin olive oil

2 tablespoons walnuts, toasted

Juice of 1 lemon

½ cup fresh basil

1 garlic clove, peeled

Pinch of sea salt

Pinch of white pepper

DIRECTIONS

Add all ingredients to a blender and puree for 2 minutes or until the mixture is smooth. Add more olive oil if necessary.

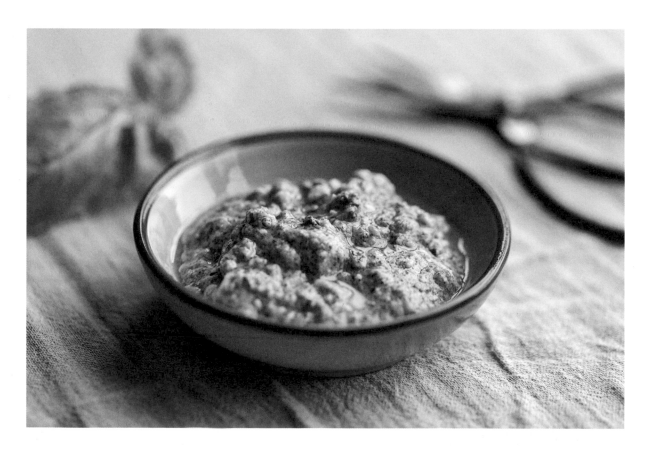

CARROT-GINGER DRESSING

Popular in Japanese restaurants, carrot-ginger dressing brings the natural sweetness of carrots together with the zesty flavor of ginger. To peel ginger quickly, cut off a chunk and take the edge of a spoon between your thumb and forefinger and work carefully in one direction to peel off the skin. It'll reveal the stringy, yellow flesh below, ready for chopping or grating.

15 MINUTES   **4** SERVINGS   VEGAN

INGREDIENTS

2 small carrots, peeled and chopped

1 tablespoon rice vinegar

½ inch ginger, peeled and mashed

1 teaspoon tamari sauce

1 teaspoon sesame oil

DIRECTIONS

1. Cook the carrots in boiling water for about 7 minutes or until they are tender. Drain the carrots.

2. Puree the carrots in a blender along with the rice vinegar, ginger, tamari sauce, and sesame oil, until the dressing is smooth but slightly granular.

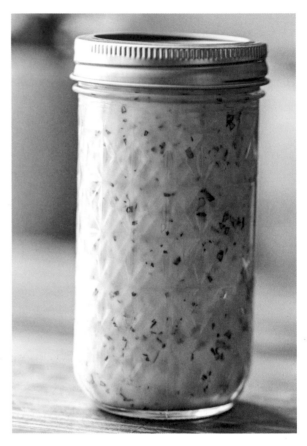

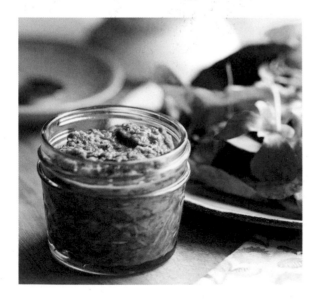

AVOCADO-CILANTRO DRESSING

If you like thick, luscious salad dressings, this one is for you. If you prefer less tanginess in your dressing or if you are adverse to dairy, then leave out the goat milk kefir—the dressing will be just as creamy without it.

15 MINUTES   **4-6** SERVINGS   VEGAN

INGREDIENTS

½ Hass avocado, mashed

2 tablespoons finely chopped cilantro

¼ cup goat milk kefir

Juice of 1 lime

2 tablespoons extra virgin olive oil

Pinch of sea salt

Pinch of white pepper

DIRECTIONS

Add all the ingredients to a mason jar. Close the jar and shake it vigorously until the dressing is creamy.

GINGER-LIME DRESSING

For a citrusy zinger, combine lime and ginger for a refreshing dressing that will jazz up any salad.

15 MINUTES   **8** SERVINGS   VEGAN

INGREDIENTS

Juice of 1 lime

2 tablespoons finely chopped cilantro

Pinch of sea salt

¼ cup extra virgin olive oil or sesame oil

1 inch ginger, peeled and minced

DIRECTIONS

Add all the ingredients to a mason jar and shake it vigorously until the dressing is well mixed.

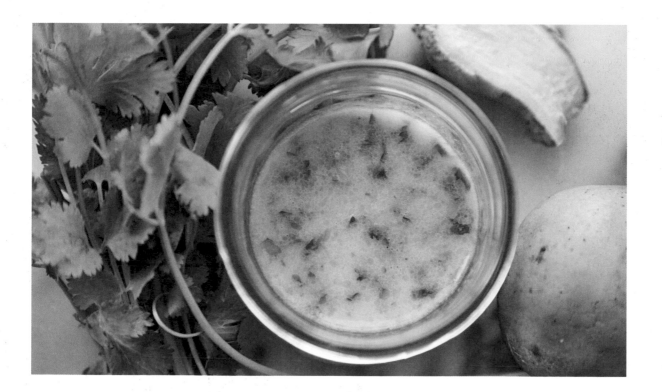

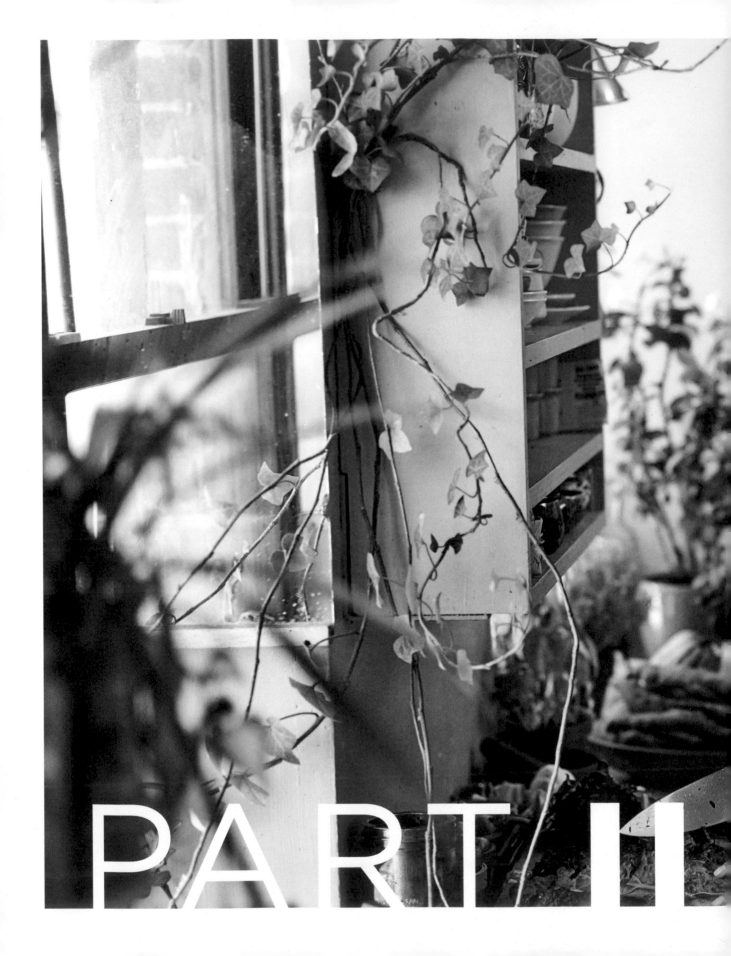

PART II

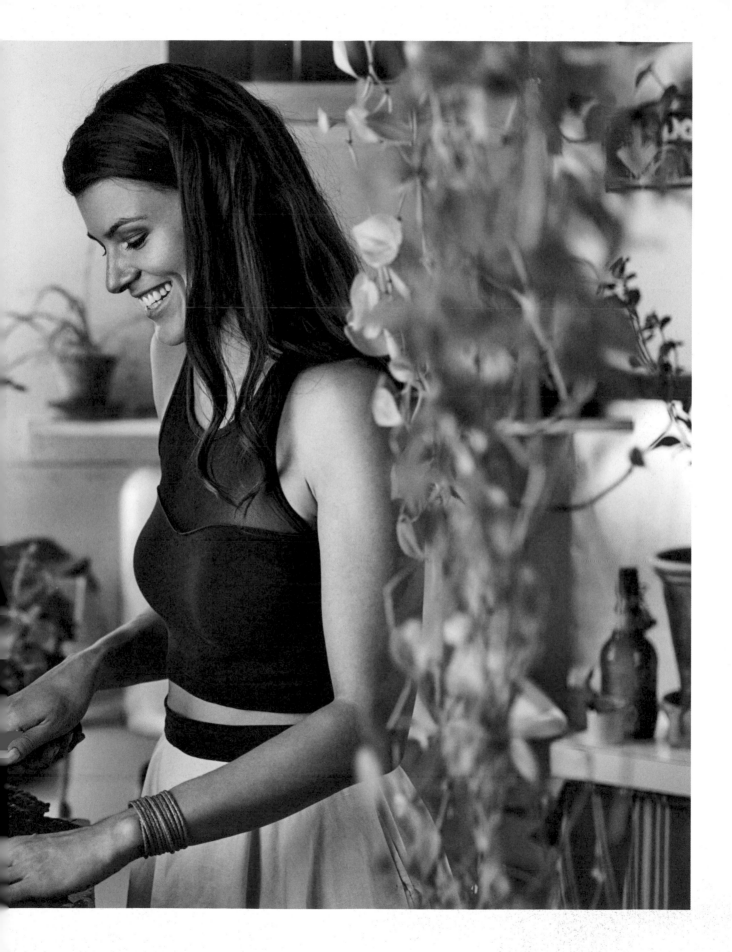

CHAPTER 5

MEAL MAPS & RECIPES

When I started my sugar detox, I knew it would be vital to plan my meals in advance. I didn't want to find myself in a grocery store deliberating what to make, because I have a tendency to browse. And when I browse, I often buy extraneous items that go to waste or, worse yet, food that isn't particularly good for me. Thus, meal planning for me doesn't begin in the grocery store or even in a recipe book. It starts with a list.

I like to buy food fresh, which means more frequent but shorter trips to the grocery store or farmers market. Given that I live in New York City, I can do that. If you live farther away from a grocery store and don't have the convenience of a grocery delivery service, then you may want to stock up on food. This is perfectly fine, but make sure you have proper storage for your fresh items so that they last longer. About one-third of the food that makes it to our homes often goes uneaten due to food spoilage and waste. This can take a bite out of your hard-earned money, so while planning your sugar detox, we might as well plan meals smartly.

I came up with the concept of Meal Maps after working with Good Eggs, a farm-to-fridge grocery delivery service. The perception is that fresh, local, organic food comes with a high price tag that is unaffordable for most people. I thought this could be resolved by showing folks that if you do some meal planning you can eat healthy, local, fresh, and even organic ingredients affordably. One night I sat down at my kitchen table and started drawing. First a whole chicken, then garlic, then an onion, kale, sweet potatoes . . . I lettered each of the items and thought about what easy meals I could make with the dozen or so ingredients I listed. Sure, I could have just written up a standard shopping list, but instead I wanted to *see* how my meals would play out over the course of 2–3 days without wasting any food. Was it possible to create a series of recipes from a dozen or so ingredients? Most certainly! It always bothered me when I would buy ingredients at the grocery store—like a bunch of asparagus—use half of it, and then forget about the other half. What a waste! Instead, I wanted to use every last bit of the food I was buying.

This is ultimately how Meal Maps developed. Meal Maps are basic plans that outline ingredients for recipes. They chart how those ingredients can be used not for only one rec-ipe but for multiple meals. Once I started to strategically plan my meals, I realized I could eat well, reduce food waste, and stay within a sensible budget—even when I wanted to buy premium products, like organic vegetables or pastured eggs, for example.

....

PLEASE NOTE: *The recipes in the Meal Maps are primarily for two people, so if you are cooking for more people or if you're an active individual with a bigger appetite, I suggest reviewing the corresponding recipes in each Meal Map; from there you can determine whether you should increase the quantity of any of the ingredients on your shopping list. Don't feel shy about eating more than one serving. These are healthy meals, so eat until you feel satisfied. And it goes without saying, if you have an allergy or an adverse reaction to any of the ingredients listed in the book, then by all means, substitute them! You know your body and appetite better than I ever will, and part of what this book is meant to do is help you rediscover the relationship you have with your body, the food you eat, and how it makes you feel.*

MEAL MAP 1

HAVE **13** PANTRY STAPLES READY AND SHOP FOR THESE **15** MAIN INGREDIENTS
TO MAKE **7** RECIPES AND **14** SERVINGS OF FOOD.

RECIPES

INGREDIENTS

1 bunch spinach

2 Hass avocados

1 bunch radishes

1 cucumber

1 bunch asparagus

5 ounces microgreen mix

2 cups sunflower or kale microgreens

2 cups mixed greens

1 bunch green onions

¾ pound tomatoes

1 bunch carrots

1 can coconut milk

10 pastured eggs

16 ounces wild-caught salmon fillet

2 slices rye or sourdough bread

PANTRY STAPLES

Shallot × 1

Fresh ginger × 1

Garlic × 1

Lemon × 2

Vegetable broth

Extra virgin olive oil

Distilled vinegar

Sherry vinegar

Salt

Pepper

Parsley

Sesame seeds

Sunflower seeds

OPTIONAL

Crushed red pepper flakes

OPTIONAL SAUCES

Hollandaise sauce

Harissa

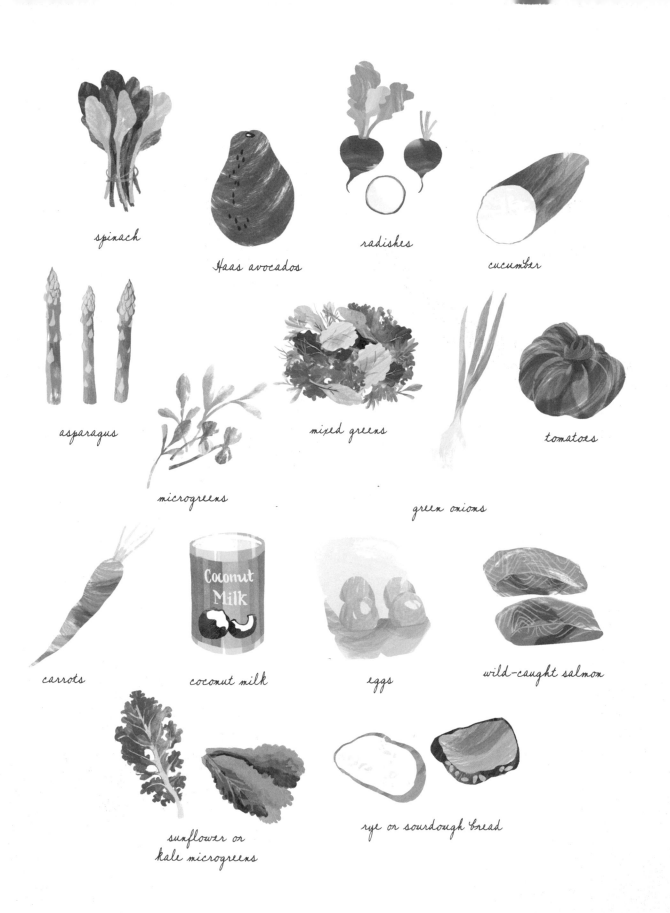

spinach

Haas avocados

radishes

cucumber

asparagus

microgreens

mixed greens

green onions

tomatoes

carrots

coconut milk

eggs

wild-caught salmon

sunflower or
kale microgreens

rye or sourdough bread

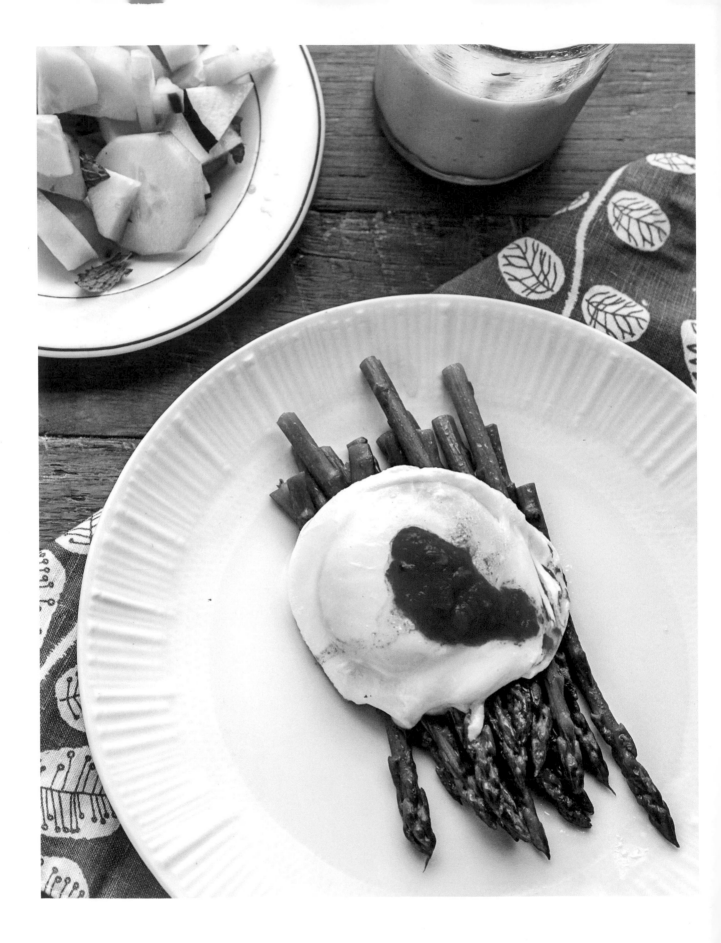

POACHED EGG OVER STEAMED ASPARAGUS WITH CUCUMBER AND RADISH SALAD

🕐 10 MINUTES   2 🍽   VEGETARIAN 🌿

When I was young, my parents raised chickens, so naturally fresh eggs were a big part of my breakfast when I was growing up. As a child my dad would ask, "How would you like your eggs?" and I would enthusiastically yell, "Sunny-side up!" I preferred them that way largely because I think I loved watching the bright yellow-orange, slightly pungent yolk (we fed the chicken marigolds) ooze out onto the plate. I didn't eat my first poached eggs, an adult version of my childhood favorite, until after college. It still oozed, but the preparation was slightly more sophisticated. Asparagus was a family favorite, too. We'd grill it, steam it, bake it, and even eat it raw. In the Northeast, asparagus and radishes are in season at about the same time, so if you can manage to find some cucumbers at the grocery store, you can have yourself a perfect breakfast: Steamed asparagus, poached egg, and a crisp, fresh side of cucumber and radish salad.

INGREDIENTS

2 eggs

2 tablespoons distilled vinegar

½ bunch asparagus

2 radishes, thinly sliced

1 cucumber, thinly sliced

¼ teaspoon sea salt

1 tablespoon sherry vinegar

Harissa (optional)

Hollandaise sauce (optional)

DIRECTIONS

1. Poach **1 egg** in water with the **distilled vinegar** in a medium saucepan for 4 minutes. Remove the egg with a slotted spoon and place it on a paper towel on a plate. Do the same for the second egg using the same water.

2. Steam the **asparagus** until it is tender. Drain and set it aside.

3. Toss the **radishes** and **cucumber** with a little **salt** and **sherry vinegar** in a small bowl. Plate them along with the **asparagus** and the **egg**. Top with **harissa** or **hollandaise sauce** for added flavor, if you like.

POACHED EGG IN AVOCADO BOAT OVER MICROGREENS

🕐 10 MINUTES   2 🍽️   VEGETARIAN 🌱

Okay, okay, so you're seeing avocados on everything—they're such an agreeable and versatile food (may you never tire of avocado toast!). The creamy, mild-tasting avocado was not a fruit that I grew up eating in northeastern Pennsylvania, because the fruits and vegetables we ate came from our garden for the most part. (I have to hand it to my mother, however, because even though nary an avocado grew in our soil, she was able to get all sorts of plants to germinate, even though their ideal growing conditions were outside of our climate zone.) Until I got to college, this pear-shaped fruit was relegated to guacamole bowls at Mexican restaurants. Avocado is particularly appetizing with eggs and greens. Just nestle a poached egg into the avocado's natural divot, where its shiny brown seed used to be. Place both halves on a bed of microgreens (a generic term for greens like lettuce, kale, and radish that unfurl their first set of leaves 1–2 weeks after germination). Microgreens are packed with nutrition and full of flavor, so I love adding them to the plate not just as "confetti" but as a central component of the meal. Plus, microgreens hold a special place in my heart because they grow extremely well indoors if you get the conditions just right, which I encourage you to try!

INGREDIENTS

2 eggs

2 tablespoons distilled vinegar

3 ounces microgreen mix

1 avocado

1 tablespoon extra virgin olive oil

¼ teaspoon sea salt

Pepper, to taste

DIRECTIONS

1. Poach **1 egg** in water with the **distilled vinegar** in medium saucepan for 4 minutes. Remove the egg with a slotted spoon and place it on a paper towel on a plate. Do the same for the second egg, using the same water.

2. Divide the **microgreens** between two plates. Halve an **avocado**, remove the pit and skin, and place each half on top of the microgreens.

3. Add a poached egg to the divot in each of the avocados. Drizzle them with **olive oil** and a sprinkling of **sea salt** and **pepper**.

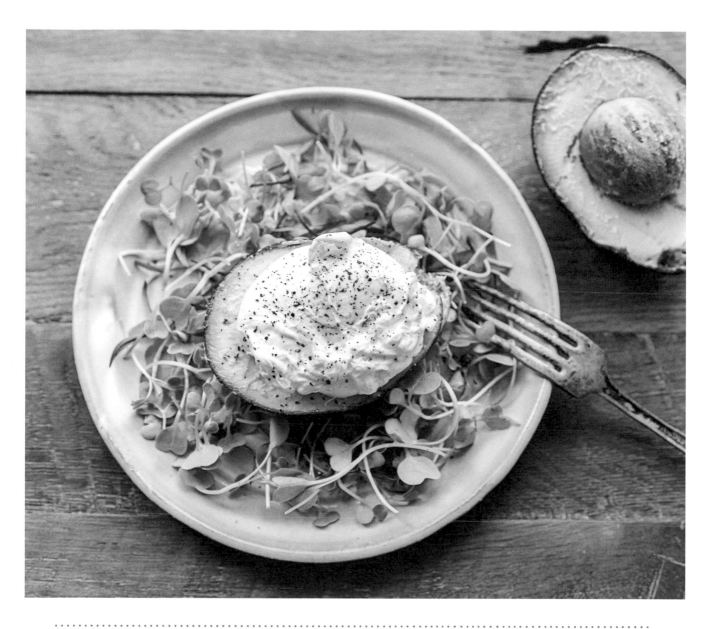

HOW TO POACH AN EGG

Get a medium-size saucepan and fill it with water about half full. Begin to simmer the water and keep it simmering. Add about 2 tablespoons of distilled vinegar to the saucepan. Crack a fresh egg into a small cup or ramekin. Begin creating a gentle whirlpool with a spoon in the simmering water. Slowly tip the ramekin or cup with the egg into the whirlpool. This helps the egg white wrap around the yolk. Leave to cook for 4 minutes. Remove egg with a slotted spoon and place on a clean kitchen towel or paper towel to remove any excess water.

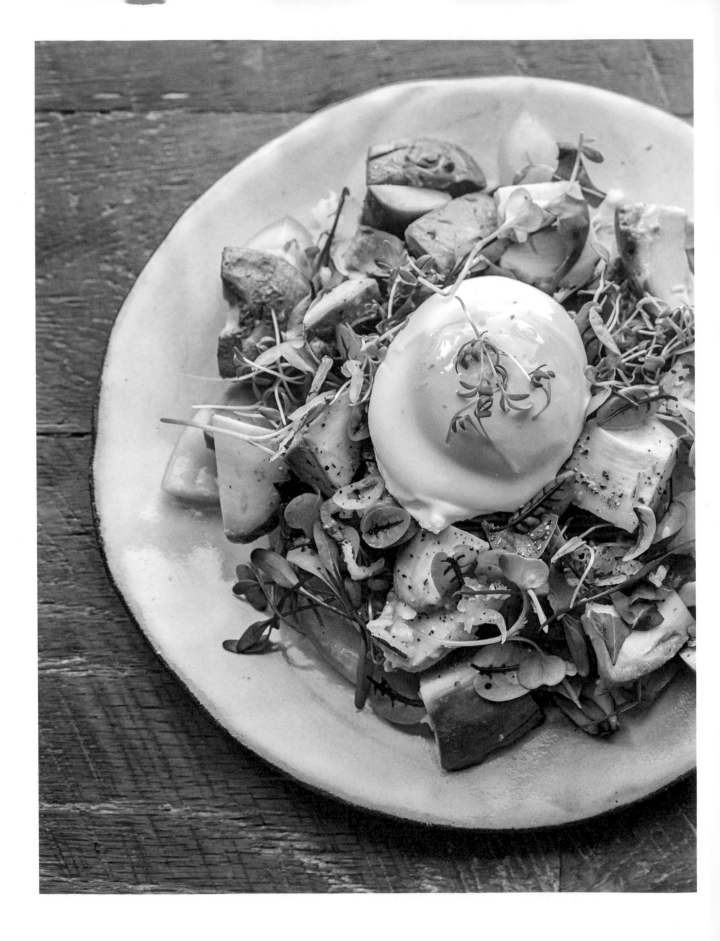

POACHED EGG OVER TOMATO AND AVOCADO SALAD

⏱ 10 MINUTES   2 🍽   VEGETARIAN 🌿

Every summer I rejoice when sun-ripened heirloom tomatoes make their debut at the farmers market. If you've only been eating conventional, flavorless beefsteak tomatoes from the grocery store, then I encourage you to try ugly but charismatic and wonderfully flavorful heirlooms. Tomatoes are rich storehouses of lycopene, a red-colored carotenoid similar to beta-carotene, but unlike beta-carotene, lycopene doesn't convert to vitamin A. Instead, it is incorporated into the small intestine. It has been shown to be beneficial for bone and cardiovascular health. Tomatoes and avocados not only taste delicious when they are paired, but also make a formidable nutritional duo. The healthy, monounsaturated fat found in avocado helps your body absorb the vitamin A you'll be getting from the tomato's other carotenoids: alpha- and beta-carotene. Add some protein by pairing the tomato and avocado with a poached egg. Vegans can substitute garbanzo beans (chickpeas) or silken tofu for the egg.

INGREDIENTS

2 eggs

2 tablespoons distilled vinegar

1 avocado, diced

1 tomato, diced

½ shallot, thinly sliced

1 ounce microgreen mix

1 tablespoon extra virgin olive oil

¼ teaspoon sea salt

Pepper, to taste

DIRECTIONS

1. Poach **1 egg** in water with the **distilled vinegar** in medium saucepan for 4 minutes. Remove the egg with a slotted spoon and place it on a paper towel on a plate. Do the same for the second egg, using the same water.

2. Plate the diced **avocado**, **tomato**, **shallots**, and **microgreens**.

3. Add a poached egg on top of the salad. Drizzle it with **olive oil** and a sprinkling of **sea salt** and **pepper**.

SPINACH AND EGG DROP SOUP

🕐 15 MINUTES   2 🍽   VEGETARIAN 🌿

For many of us, our first taste of egg drop soup came from a plastic container along with a fortune cookie, duck sauce, and white rice. I began making my own version with tatsoi, which is a firm, spinach-like plant with a mild, mustardy bite. This recipe calls for spinach because it's easier to find in most markets, but if you're able to locate some tatsoi, then I encourage you to be adventurous and swap it in as the main green. You'll be surprised how easy this soup is to make. Within seconds of adding the egg, the broth thickens, and moments later, you'll be ladling the sumptuous mixture into a bowl, never to return to Chinese takeout. How's that for a fortune, sans cookie?

INGREDIENTS

1 tablespoon extra virgin olive oil

½ shallot, thinly sliced

1 tablespoon peeled and julienned ginger

2 cloves garlic, chopped

4 cups vegetable broth, store-bought, or use the recipe for Homemade Vegetable Broth that follows

Pinch sea salt, to taste

Pepper, to taste

2 eggs, lightly beaten

1 bunch spinach

Handful green onion, chopped

Parsley

¼ teaspoon sesame seeds

DIRECTIONS

1. Heat the **olive oil** in a deep pot over medium heat and add the **shallot** and **ginger**, stirring for about 2 minutes until they are fragrant. Add the **garlic** and sauté for another minute.

2. Pour the **vegetable broth** (or you can use water) over the shallot and garlic mixture. Season with **salt** and **pepper**. Bring to a simmer.

3. Whisk the **eggs** in a small bowl with a little salt and pepper.

4. Add the **spinach** and **green onions** to the vegetable broth and cook until wilted, about 30 seconds. Begin stirring in the egg mixture slowly. Season to taste, garnish, and serve.

HOMEMADE VEGETABLE BROTH

2 garlic cloves, sliced

½ yellow onion, diced

1 tablespoon extra virgin olive oil

2–3 carrots, diced

1–2 carrot tops

2 celery stalks

2–4 sprigs thyme

16 cups water

1–2 bay leaves, optional

1 teaspoon celery seeds, optional

1–2 cloves, optional

1. Sauté the garlic and onion with the olive oil in the bottom of a pressure cooker until they are fragrant, approximately 2 minutes.

2. Add the remainder of the ingredients to the pressure cooker. Use at least 16 cups of water or fill the cooker ¾ of the way full. Seal the pressure cooker, bring it to pressure, and cook for 50 minutes.

3. Turn off the heat. The pressure will drop automatically. Strain the liquid through a sieve into another large pot. I often also use a heavy duty paper towel with the sieve as well. Press the liquid from the vegetables into the new pot. Compost the remaining vegetables.

4. Use the Homemade Vegetable Broth for the various soups or sauces in this book.

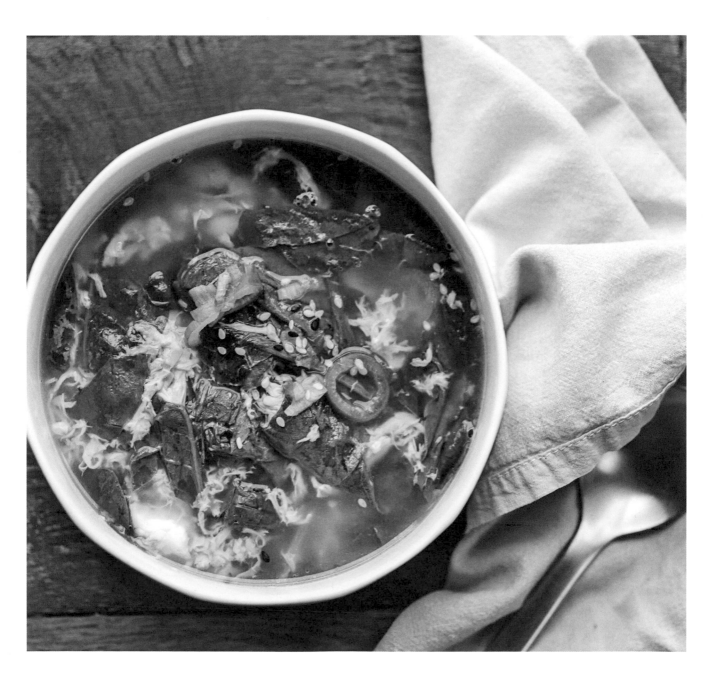

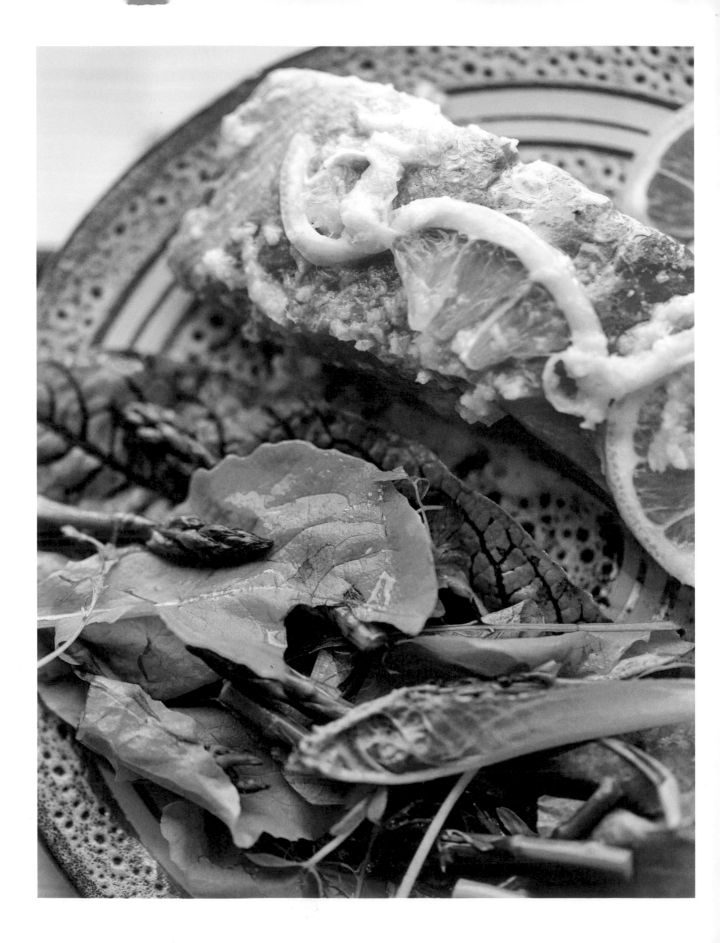

GINGERED SALMON WITH ASPARAGUS AND MIXED GREENS

30 MINUTES   **2**   **PESCATARIAN**

Many folks I know who claim to not like fish often follow up with the non sequitur "but I eat salmon." Everyone seems to have his or her own reason for loving salmon: It's meaty and flavorful, yet not too fishy, or it's a superfood. In fact, salmon is all of those things—if you're able to nab a wild-caught fish during the peak season (May to October), that is. When I buy salmon, I often opt for wild-caught salmon from the Pacific Northwest, for which I have a newfound appreciation after spending time in British Columbia during the salmon runs (and catching one with my bare hands—*for real!*). You may find delightful salmon varieties behind the fish counter—coho, king, chum, and sockeye—and all of them have subtly different flavors and textures. King is particularly expensive, but since I don't recommend eating fish every day, I would encourage you to treat yourself and notice the distinct flavor and difference in texture between a wild-caught and farm-raised salmon. Adding some simple steamed asparagus and salad greens will make this a well-earned meal, particularly after a hard workout.

INGREDIENTS

2 8-ounce wild-caught salmon fillets

1 lemon

¼ teaspoon pureed ginger

⅛ teaspoon sea salt

1 teaspoon pepper

1½ tablespoons extra virgin olive oil, divided

½ bunch asparagus

2 cups mixed greens

½–1 lemon, thinly sliced (optional)

DIRECTIONS

1. Preheat the oven to 400°F. Place the **salmon** fillets in a glass baking dish.

2. Cut the **lemon** in half and juice it into a small bowl.

3. Add the **ginger**, **salt**, and **pepper** to the bowl with the lemon juice and add 1 tablespoon of the **olive oil**. Mix well. Pour generously over the salmon fillets.

4. Bake the salmon fillets for 15 minutes, ensuring they flake well with a fork.

5. Steam the **asparagus** until it is tender. Combine with the **mixed greens.**

6. Plate the asparagus and greens. Drizzle the remaining olive oil over the top along with a sprinkle of salt. Add the salmon and serve. Garnish with lemon slices, if desired.

CHOOSING FISH

When shopping for fish, always aim to get wild-caught, sustainably harvested fish from a trusted fishmonger whenever possible. I know it's more expensive than farmed fish, but wild-caught fish are more often than not eating wild things, like algae and smaller fish. Not all farmed fish eat the same thing, but farmed herbivorous fish typically eat soy and corn, which is most likely genetically modified, and carnivorous fish are typically eating a protein/fish oil/plant pellet. Remember, you are what you eat and what your food eats, so you'll want to eat a fish that has eaten a healthier, more balanced diet so that you can get all the benefits, particularly those omega-3 fatty acids.

You will likely want to limit your fish intake to no more than 2 pounds per week. Why? Nearly all fish contain trace amounts of methylmercury, largely caused by manmade pollution in the atmosphere. Larger predatory fish, which feed on other fish, bioaccumulate more methylmercury than herbivorous fish, or bottom feeders, like mussels and clams. Try to have fish like swordfish or warm-water tuna no more than once a month, and not at all if you are a pregnant woman or thinking of becoming pregnant.

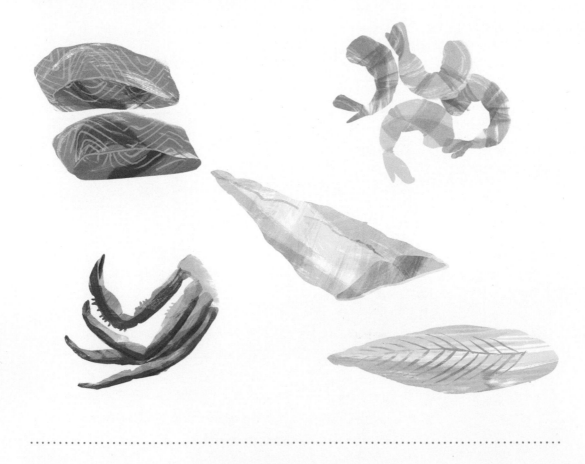

CARROT-TOMATO SOUP

🕐 20 MINUTES　　2 🍽　　VEGAN ✕

Tomatoes were a mainstay when I was a kid, because during the height of the season, from mid-June through October, they were plentiful. And, as wasting any food was forbidden, my grandparents and parents had an arsenal of tomato recipes to draw on: stewed tomatoes, pickled tomatoes, homemade tomato sauce, and of course tomato soup. Carrots in the Northeast conveniently overlap with tomato season and add a sweet, rooty goodness to the soup. Though it was traditional to use heavy cream or whole milk in our creamy soup recipes, I've found coconut milk to be a delicious substitute, particularly if you use the first inch of coconut cream that often forms near the top of the can. Top this soup with microgreens and sop it up with some fresh-baked sourdough bread.

INGREDIENTS

1 tablespoon extra virgin olive oil

2 garlic cloves, minced

1 can coconut milk

1 cup pureed tomatoes

2 cups chopped carrots

¼ teaspoon sea salt, to taste

Pinch of pepper, to taste

1 tablespoon microgreens (optional)

DIRECTIONS

1. Heat the **olive oil** in a medium saucepan and add the **garlic**. Sauté the garlic for about 1 minute or until it is fragrant.

2. Add the **remaining ingredients** to the saucepan and bring to a boil. Turn heat down and let the mixture cook for 15 minutes.

3. Remove the saucepan from the heat. Puree the mixture using an immersion blender or let it cool and blend in a blender. Pour the soup into bowls, garnish with **microgreens**, and serve warm.

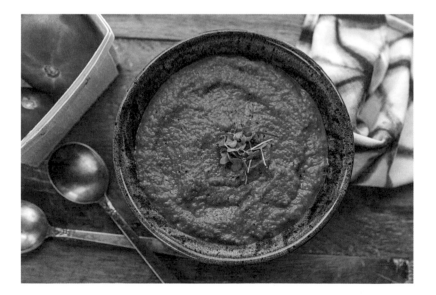

SUNFLOWER GREENS AND RADISH SALAD WITH A SUNNY-SIDE UP EGG

🕐 25 MINUTES   2 🍽   VEGETARIAN 🌱

The crunch of sunflower greens and radishes doesn't need to be reserved just for salads. You can create a perfect little meal by adding them to a slice of toast, topped with a sunny-side up egg and sprinkled with whatever leftover greens and lemon juice you may have on hand. Keeping everything on the bread and the yolk from dripping on your chin requires another skill set altogether—one that I've yet to master!

INGREDIENTS

1½ tablespoons extra virgin olive oil, divided

2 eggs

½ cup radishes, thinly sliced

2 cups sunflower and/or kale microgreens

2 tablespoons lemon juice

Pinch of sea salt

Pinch of pepper

2 slices rye or sourdough bread

¼ cup sunflower seeds

Crushed red pepper flakes (optional)

DIRECTIONS

1. Heat 1 tablespoon of the **olive oil** in a nonstick skillet over medium heat. Crack two **eggs** into the skillet and cover it. Let the eggs steam for 2–3 minutes, making sure not to overcook the yolks.

2. While the eggs are steaming, place the **radishes** and **microgreens** in a bowl. Toss them with the remaining ½ tablespoon of olive oil, the **lemon juice**, and the **salt** and **pepper**.

3. Toast the **bread**. Place half of the greens and one of the eggs on top of each slice of toast. Sprinkle with half of the **sunflower seeds** and some **crushed red pepper flakes**, if you have them. Enjoy.

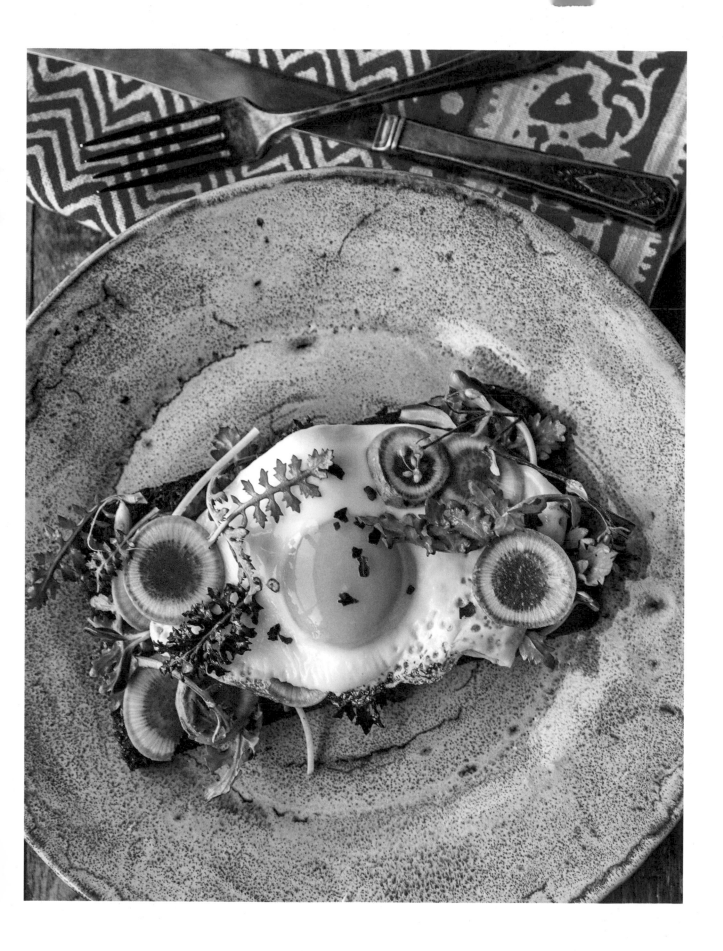

MEAL MAP 2

HAVE **14** PANTRY STAPLES READY, SHOP FOR THESE **13** MAIN INGREDIENTS, AND MAKE **7** RECIPES AND **23** SERVINGS.

RECIPES

INGREDIENTS

1 butternut squash

2 sweet potatoes

4 small red potatoes

1½ bunches kale

3 cups Lacinato kale

1 pound Brussels sprouts

3 ounces microgreens (pea tendril, or your choice)

1 tomato

2 celery stalks

1 bunch carrots

6 pastured eggs

1 whole chicken

1 pound spicy chorizo

PANTRY STAPLES

Sweet yellow onion × 2

Lemon × 2

Garlic × 1

Vegetable or chicken broth

Extra virgin olive oil

Distilled vinegar

Salt

Pepper

Paprika

Cayenne pepper

Cloves

Celery seeds

Bay leaves

Thyme

OPTIONAL SAUCES

Avocado-Cilantro Dressing

OPTIONAL

Crushed red pepper

Green onion

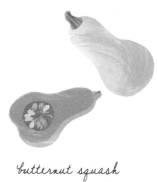

butternut squash

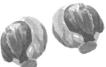

sweet potatoes

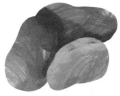

red potatoes

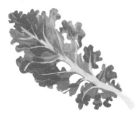

kale

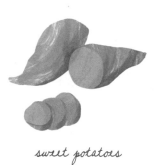

Lacinato kale

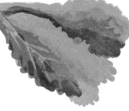

Brussels sprouts

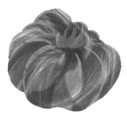

tomato

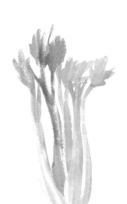

celery stalks

carrots

microgreens (pea tendril, or your choice)

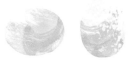

eggs

whole chicken

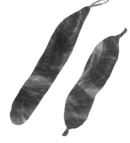

spicy chorizo

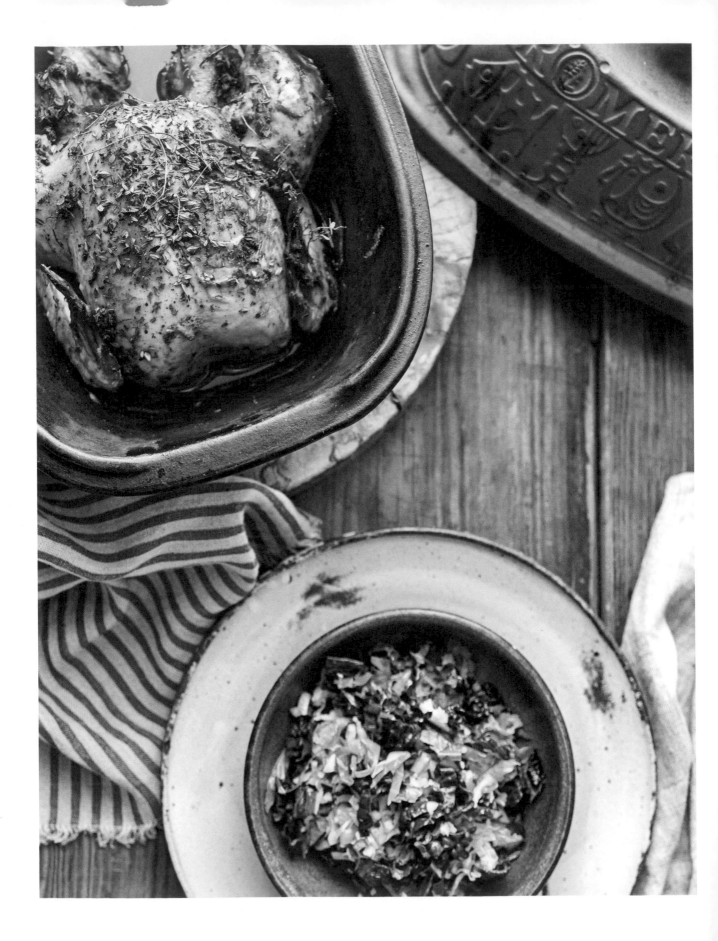

OVEN-ROASTED SPICED CHICKEN WITH A SIDE OF SHAVED BRUSSELS SPROUTS AND KALE SALAD

● ⏱ 75 MINUTES   🍽 3   NON-VEGETARIAN 🍴

For the last year or so, with some exceptions, I've been implementing a "meat only on Mondays" policy (as opposed to a "meatless Monday"), which is a symbolic reminder that we should all eat more veggies. Though I'm personally cooking less with meat, one of my all-time favorite dishes is a whole organic chicken, marinated in herbs and spices and roasted in a clay pot. This method keeps the chicken mouthwateringly succulent while simultaneously crisping the outside skin to a glorious golden-brown. You'll want to check the chicken halfway through the cooking time to make sure there is enough juice from the chicken to steam it in the clay pot. If it looks a little dry, just add a bit of water to moisten as it cooks. Give yourself a large helping of the kale and Brussels sprouts salad, and you'll have yourself a meal, along with some leftovers if you're only cooking for one or two.

INGREDIENTS

1 whole chicken (3 pounds)

2 teaspoons sea salt

1 teaspoon pepper

1 tablespoon paprika

1 teaspoon cayenne

2 tablespoons extra virgin olive oil, divided

2 cups kale, ribboned

½ pound Brussels sprouts, ribboned

1 lemon

DIRECTIONS

1. Preheat the oven to 375°F. Wash the whole **chicken** and rub in the **salt**, **pepper**, **paprika**, and **cayenne**. I prefer to cook my chicken in a covered clay pot to retain moisture, but you can cook it in a glass pan covered with aluminum foil. Add 1 tablespoon of the **olive oil** and a little water, if necessary, to add moisture. Cook for 60–70 minutes.

2. Wash your hands thoroughly with soap and water after handling the chicken. Add the **kale**, **Brussels sprouts**, the remaining 1 tablespoon of the olive oil, and some salt and pepper to a bowl. Zest a **lemon**; set the zest aside, juice the lemon, and add the lemon juice to the mixture. Massage it thoroughly into the kale and Brussels sprouts until the leaves are softened.

3. Remove the chicken from the oven. Plate the shaved Brussels sprouts and kale salad, and add the lemon zest to the top. Serve.

HOMEMADE CHICKEN BROTH

● 60 MINUTES   🍽 8   NON-VEGETARIAN 🍴🍽

One of the many benefits of roasting a whole chicken is being able to make a warm, comforting broth from the bones and any remaining veggie offcuts (onion skins included, which are particularly nutritious). To make this broth, it's ideal to have 3–4 pounds of bones, which you can collect, wrap, and freeze over time until you're ready to get your broth on, but I also make a more diluted chicken stock from the bones of one whole roasted chicken from a previous meal. I then use the broth to make soups or to simmer pulses, like beans and lentils, to give them additional flavor. Any leftover broth can be frozen, but the key to freezing is to fill BPA-free containers at most three-quarters full and freezing it *before* capping the container. Liquid expands when it freezes, so if you put on the lid beforehand, it'll likely crack the container and you'll have a bit of a mess in your freezer. It's best to put the top on only when the broth is fully frozen.

INGREDIENTS

2 garlic cloves, peeled and sliced

½ yellow onion, diced

1 tablespoon extra virgin olive oil

2–3 carrots, diced

1–2 carrot tops

2 celery stalks

2–4 sprigs of thyme

Chicken bones

1–2 bay leaves

1 tablespoon celery seeds

1–2 cloves

16 cups water

DIRECTIONS

1. Sauté the **garlic** and **onion** in the **olive oil** in the bottom of a pressure cooker for about 2 minutes or until the veggies are fragrant.

2. Add the **remainder of the ingredients** to the pressure cooker. Use at least 16 cups of **water** or fill three-quarters of the way full. Seal the pressure cooker, bring to pressure, and cook for 40–50 minutes.

3. Turn off the heat. The pressure will drop automatically. Strain the liquid through a sieve into another large pot. I often use a heavy-duty paper towel with the sieve as well. Press the liquid from the veggies into the new pot. Compost the remaining vegetables.

4. Use the chicken broth to make **Azorean Kale Soup** in Meal Map 2, Recipe 3, or in other soups or sauces. Freeze the remaining broth for up to 6 months.

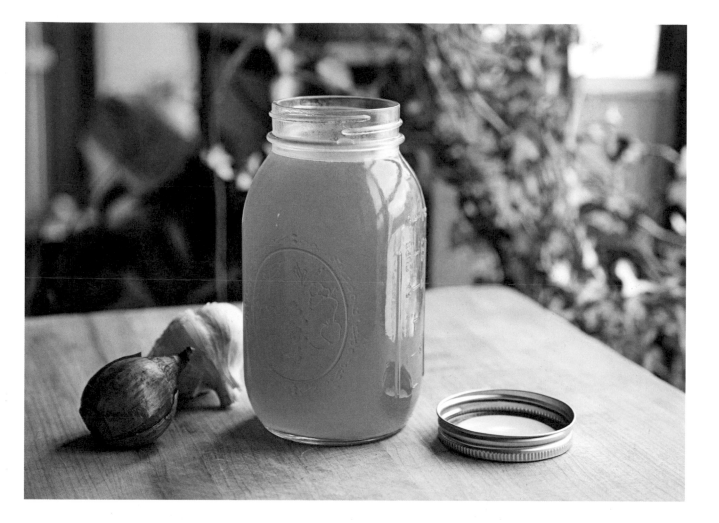

COMPOSTING

I grew up in northeastern Pennsylvania. Composting was natural there. Food turns into soil when it decomposes; why waste perfectly fine resources? In New York City, where I live now, I've been a big advocate for curbside organics pickup, but in the meantime, I keep my compost in the freezer and take it out weekly to the farmers market, where it gets turned into compost that you can purchase or that is used in community gardens around the city. When cooking at home, I encourage anyone— no matter where they are—to begin composting. It reduces waste considerably and helps give back much-needed nutrients to our food system.

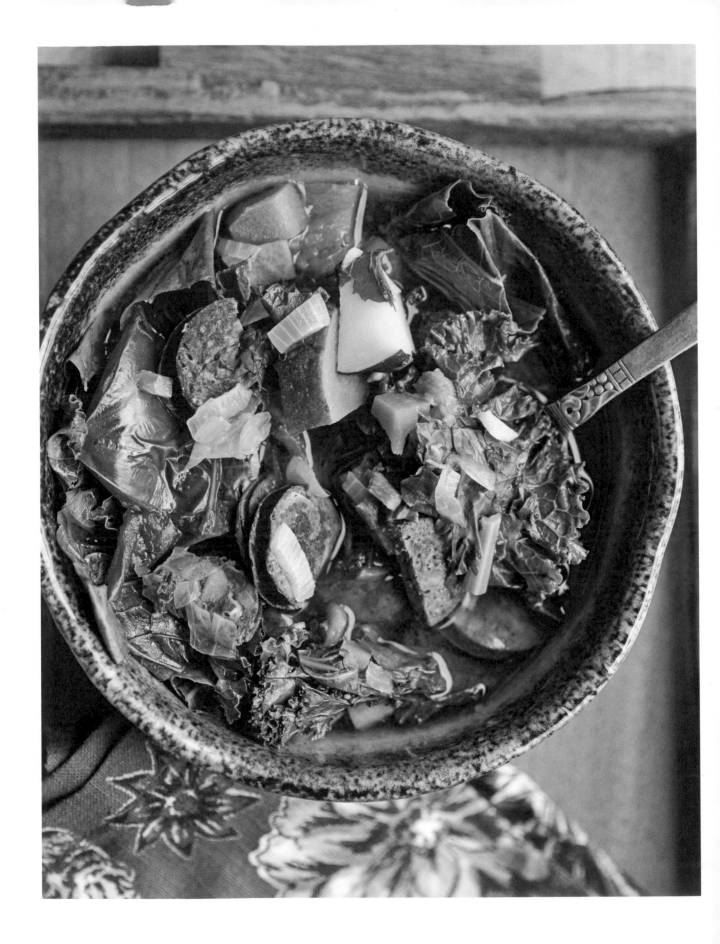

AZOREAN KALE SOUP

🕐 35 MINUTES   4 🍽   NON-VEGETARIAN 🍴

INGREDIENTS

2 tablespoons extra virgin olive oil

4 small red potatoes, diced

1 sweet potato, diced

½ butternut squash, peeled, deseeded, and diced

1 large yellow onion, chopped

2-4 garlic cloves, diced

1 bay leaf

1 bunch fresh kale, washed, destemmed, and shredded

½ teaspoon sea salt

⅛ teaspoon ground black pepper

1 tomato, diced

½ pound spicy chorizo (omit if vegetarian)

2 quarts chicken (or vegetable) broth, store-bought, or use the recipe for Homemade Chicken Broth on page 78 (or Homemade Vegetable Broth on page 66)

I first made this soup for my best friend, Paul, whose family is from the Azores, an idyllic archipelago just 845 miles west of Portugal. I only see Paul once or twice a year, so when he comes to New York, it's a real treat. I decided to cook him something that would remind him a bit of his family's homeland. Azorean kale soup is traditionally made with linguiça, a smoked sausage, but it can also be made with a spicy chorizo or spicy kielbasa. Even without the meat, however, the soup is comforting and hearty, thanks to the addition of potatoes and squash. Vegetarians can also substitute beans for the meat. Add a little extra heat and savory flavor by adding some chiles and smoked paprika to the mix.

DIRECTIONS

1. Heat the **olive oil** in a deep pot or pressure cooker over medium-high heat. Add the **potatoes, sweet potato, butternut squash,** and **onions.** Cover and cook for 5 minutes, stirring if necessary.

2. Add the **garlic, bay leaf,** and **kale.** Cover for about 2 minutes or until the kale is wilted. Add **salt** and **pepper.**

3. Add the **tomato,** the **chorizo,** and the **broth.** Bring to a boil, and then reduce heat and simmer for 20 minutes. If you are using a pressure cooker, bring to pressure for 5-8 minutes. Serve.

BUTTERNUT SQUASH AND KALE SALAD WITH AVOCADO-CILANTRO DRESSING

🕐 40 MINUTES   2 🍽   VEGETARIAN 🌿

The sweet, buttery flavor and firm yet creamy texture of butternut squash pairs nicely with the bitter, crisp bite of massaged Lacinato kale in this salad. The velvety texture of the avocado-cilantro dressing coats the pebbly texture of this *Brassica*—and if you like heavy, creamy dressings, you can serve yourself a lot of this one! The added nutritional benefits of this dish are undeniable: 1 cup of butternut squash provides nearly 7 grams of fiber (about one-quarter of the suggested daily intake of fiber for women); tons of vitamins A, C, and B_6; magnesium; potassium; and more. To top it off, 1 cup of fresh kale will give you an additional 0.6 grams of fiber and additional boosts of vitamins C and B_6, potassium, and alpha-lipoic acid, which has been shown to positively increase insulin sensitivity in the body. Half an avocado has 6 grams of fiber, vitamin K, and a host of phytochemicals. To sum it up, one serving of this salad will give you about half of the suggested daily fiber intake, if you're a woman, and about a third, if you're a man. You might as well help yourself to another serving if you're hungry!

INGREDIENTS

½ butternut squash, peeled, deseeded, and diced

2 tablespoons extra virgin olive oil, divided

2 cups Lacinato kale, ribboned

Sea salt, to taste

Pepper, to taste

Juice of 1 lemon (optional)

Crushed red pepper (optional)

Avocado-Cilantro Dressing (optional; see recipe on page 52)

DIRECTIONS

1. Toss the **butternut squash** in a large bowl with 1 tablespoon of the **olive oil**.

2. Preheat the oven to 350°F. Spread the butternut squash on a baking sheet and bake for about 30 minutes, turning the squash about halfway through. Remove the squash from the oven.

3. Place the **kale** in a large bowl and add the remaining tablespoon of olive oil, **salt**, and **pepper** and massage the kale thoroughly until it becomes supple. Use the **lemon juice** as well, if you have it handy, but it's not necessary.

4. Toss the butternut squash in with the kale. Add **crushed red pepper**, if you like, and toss with a **homemade dressing**. I suggest **Avocado-Cilantro Dressing**.

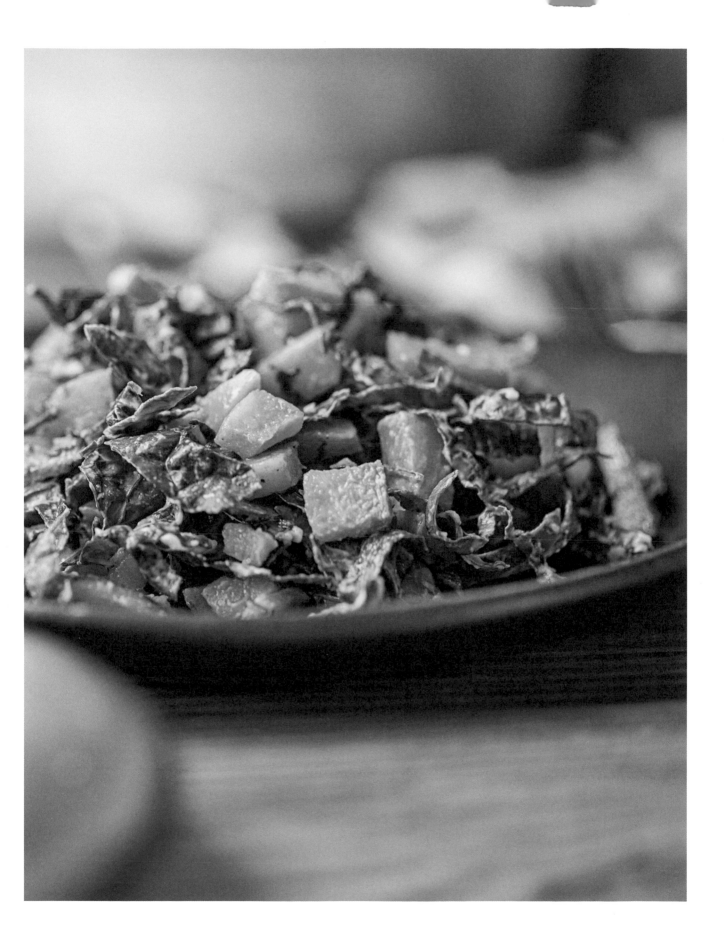

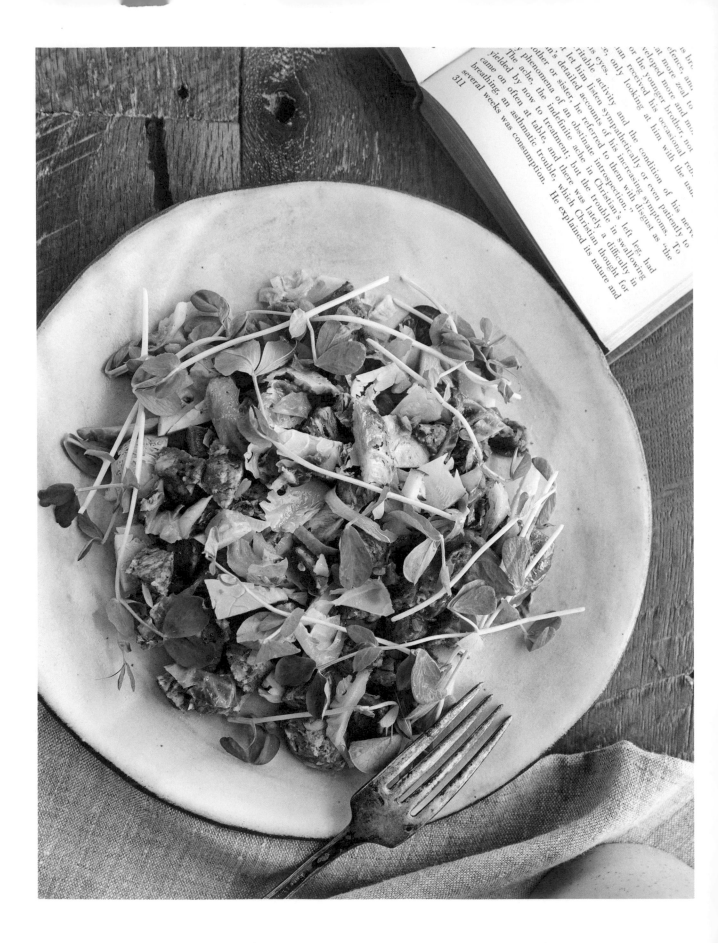

SAUTÉED BRUSSELS SPROUTS WITH CHORIZO

🕐 10 MINUTES   2 🍽   NON-VEGETARIAN 🍴

Brussels sprouts, which look like miniature cabbages, grow on a thick green stalk. Though we commonly just eat the sprout, the stalk—which is chock-full of fiber and phytonutrients—is edible, too, but it requires a lot more steaming and work. If you want to keep it easy on yourself, just pick up some Brussels sprouts at the farmers market or grocery store. Vegans and vegetarians can substitute tempeh for the chorizo sausage.

INGREDIENTS

1 tablespoon extra virgin olive oil

½ pound Brussels sprouts, ribboned

2 chorizo links, diced

3 ounces microgreens (pea tendril, or your choice)

Sea Salt, to taste

Pepper, to taste

DIRECTIONS

1. Heat the **olive oil** in a nonstick skillet over medium heat. Add the **Brussels sprouts** and sauté them for 1 minute. Add the **chorizo** and cook for 2–3 more minutes.

2. Plate the Brussels sprouts and chorizo mixture, and add the **microgreens**. Season with **salt** and **pepper**, as needed.

POACHED EGG OVER SWEET POTATO HASH

🕐 10 MINUTES   2 🍽   VEGETARIAN 🫛

Sweet potatoes, particularly with their skin on, provide an excellent source of fiber—half a spud will give you around 3 grams and a significant dose of vitamin A, potassium, and choline. Choline is absolutely vital for methylation, which is important for many of our basic cellular processes, including liver detoxification. There are many varieties of sweet potatoes. I've found that sweet potatoes with creamy flesh are mild, the orange ones are sweet, and purple sweet potatoes are so much like candy that I've even eaten them as a dessert! Add a poached or sunny-side up pastured egg (also rich in choline!) to this delicious hash and notice how well-balanced your blood sugar will be until your next meal.

INGREDIENTS

2 eggs

2 tablespoons distilled vinegar

1 tablespoon extra virgin olive oil

1 sweet potato, cut into matchstick-size pieces

Sea salt, to taste

Pepper, to taste

Green onion (optional)

DIRECTIONS

1. Poach **1 egg** in water with the **distilled vinegar** in medium saucepan for 4 minutes. Remove the egg with a slotted spoon and place it on a paper towel on a plate. Do the same for the second egg, using the same water.

2. Heat the **olive oil** in a nonstick skillet and sauté the **sweet potato** over medium-high heat for 5 minutes, stirring regularly so the potatoes don't burn or stick to the bottom of the pan. Add **salt** and **pepper**. Continue to cook the potatoes on a lower temperature, if you like them crispy.

3. Plate the potatoes. Chop a **green onion**, if you have one, and sprinkle it over the poached egg. Serve.

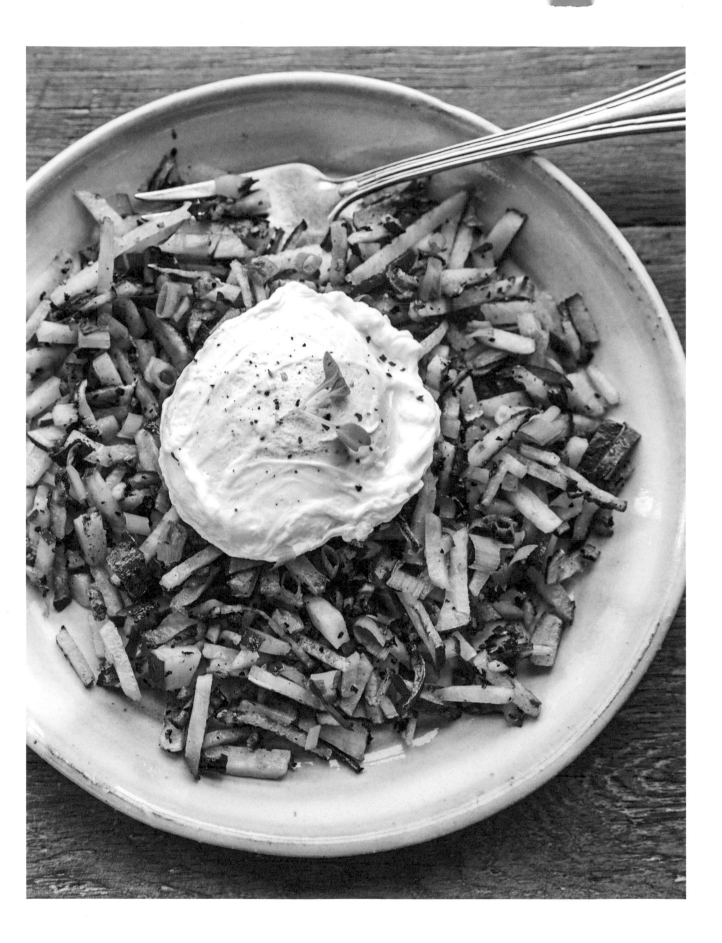

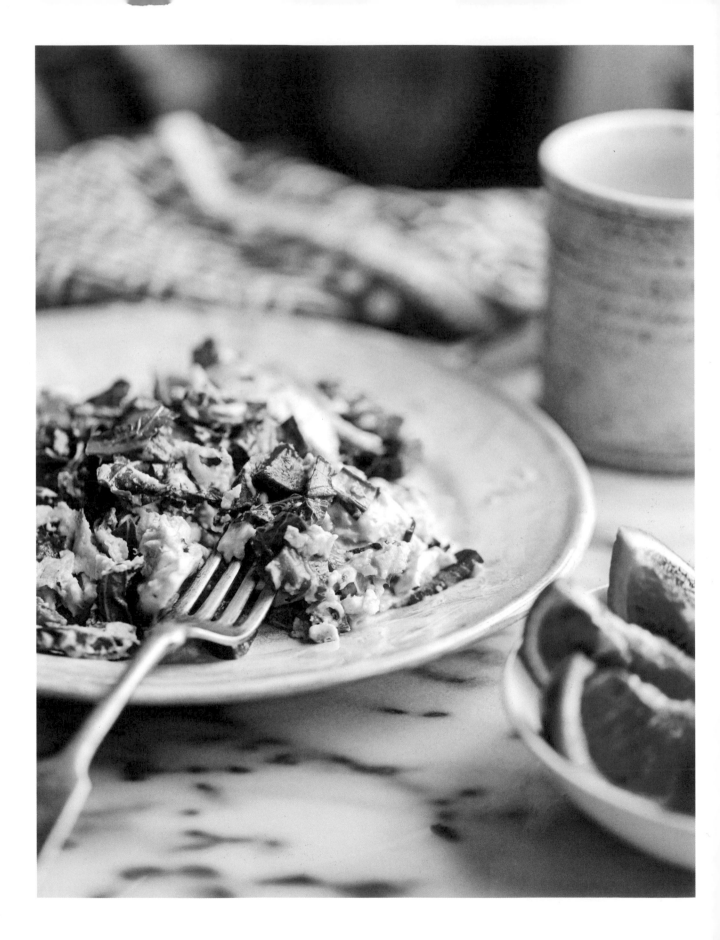

EGG, KALE, AND CHORIZO SCRAMBLE

10 MINUTES   2   NON-VEGETARIAN

It may be surprising, but our bodies can produce all the necessary fuel we need from both protein and fat, and this dish serves up both. The egg and chorizo in this dish provide a protein-rich breakfast, so if you're planning to have a long break between breakfast and lunch, this will surely keep you satisfied in the meantime without spiking your insulin and therefore reducing any temptation for snacking.

INGREDIENTS

4 eggs

1 tablespoon extra virgin olive oil

2 chorizo links, sliced

1 cup Lacinato kale, washed, destemmed, and chopped

Pinch sea salt

Pinch black pepper

DIRECTIONS

1. Crack the **eggs** into a bowl and stir until beaten.

2. Heat the **olive oil** in a nonstick skillet over medium heat; add the eggs. Heat for about 1 minute. As the egg starts to firm, add the **chorizo**. Place a lid on the skillet and let the eggs heat for another minute. Then add the **kale** and let it steam for about 2 minutes.

3. Use a spatula to break up the eggs and scramble them. Taste and add more **salt** or **pepper** to your liking.

MEAL MAP 3

HAVE 17 PANTRY STAPLES READY AND SHOP FOR THESE 17 MAIN INGREDIENTS TO MAKE 8 RECIPES AND 24 SERVINGS.

RECIPES

INGREDIENTS

3 pounds mixed mushrooms

13 portobello mushroom caps

½ pound cremini mushrooms

1 bunch leeks

3 scallions

1¼ pounds carrots

1 pound Brussels sprouts

1 bok choy

1 bunch curly kale

2 bunches arugula or other salad greens

1 avocado

1 bunch celery stalks

2 radishes

2 large artichokes

6 pastured eggs

2 whole organic chicken breasts

PANTRY STAPLES

Salt

Pepper

Yellow onion × 2

Shallot × 6

Garlic × 1

Lemon × 2

Ginger × 1

Pearl barley

Extra virgin olive oil

Ghee

Coconut flour

Parsley

Bay leaves

Thyme

Balsamic vinegar

SAUCES

Tamari

Aioli

OPTIONAL

Scallion microgreens

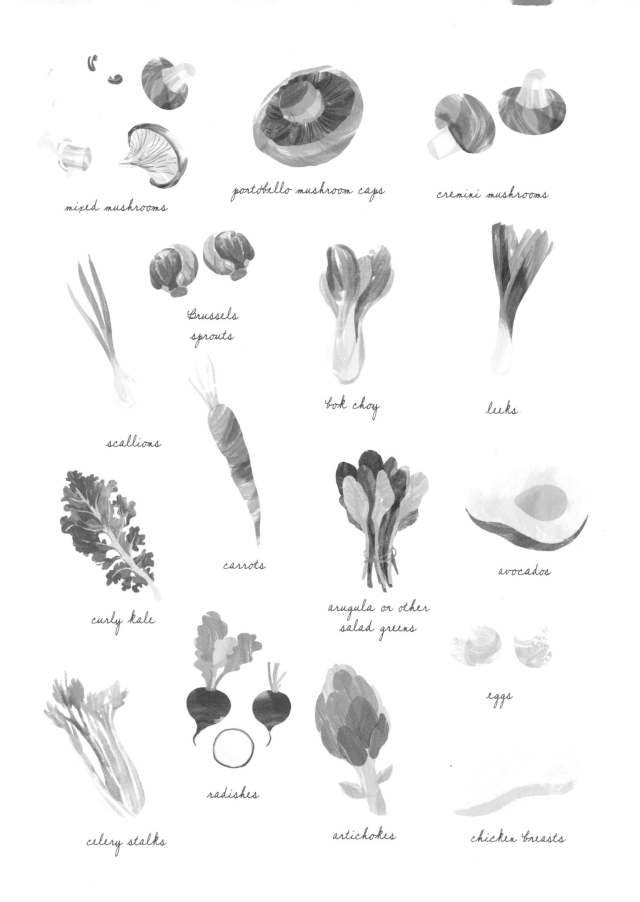

mixed mushrooms

portobello mushroom caps

cremini mushrooms

Brussels sprouts

bok choy

leeks

scallions

carrots

avocados

curly kale

arugula or other salad greens

eggs

celery stalks

radishes

artichokes

chicken breasts

MUSHROOM BROTH

● 🕐 75 MINUTES   6 🍽   VEGAN 🍴

As a young girl I would venture into the forest near my home and collect and document fungi. It was in eighth grade biology class with my teacher Mr. Alessio that my love of mushrooms really started to flourish and, for a while, I flirted with the idea of becoming a mycologist. In college I took a rather infamous class with Professor George Hudler titled *Magical Mushrooms, Mischievous Molds*, which further opened a Pandora's box of curiosity and taste for mushrooms; it was with that class that I first ate the delicate flesh of a morel and sipped on the highly appetizing (but strangely unappealing-looking) corn smut or Huitlacoche soup. Mushrooms and their health properties are so unique that I always felt they should be in a class—or at least a food group—all of their own. Mushrooms are rich in antioxidants and an incredible source of selenium, vitamin D, and folate. Grab a handful of the most common mushrooms—buttons, bellas, and oysters—and turn them into a stock the same way you would vegetable or chicken broth. The 'shrooms bring out an earthy, meaty umami flavor and are perfect for making myriad dishes, from savory "oats" to belly-warming soups.

INGREDIENTS

2 pounds mushrooms or mushroom trimmings (e.g., button, bella, and oyster mushrooms, or whatever variety you have on hand)

1 large yellow onion, halved

1 celery stalk, chopped

1 carrot, chopped

2 cloves garlic

1 bay leaf

A few sprigs of thyme

A few sprigs of parsley

¼ teaspoon salt

⅛ teaspoon pepper

12 cups water

DIRECTIONS

1. Toss **all the ingredients** into a large pot with about 12 cups of **water** or up to the line a pressure cooker. If you're using a pressure cooker, set it on high and then reduce to low. Bring the ingredients to a simmer for about 1 hour or longer.

2. Strain the broth. I use a fine-mesh sieve with a paper towel placed on the inside.

NOTE: *Mushrooms have a tendency to hold a lot of water, so make sure you press down on them to get out all the good juices.*

NOTE: *I've found that the mushrooms stay flavorful, even after pressing, so I use them in other recipes—Chicken with Sautéed Mushrooms (page 99), for example.*

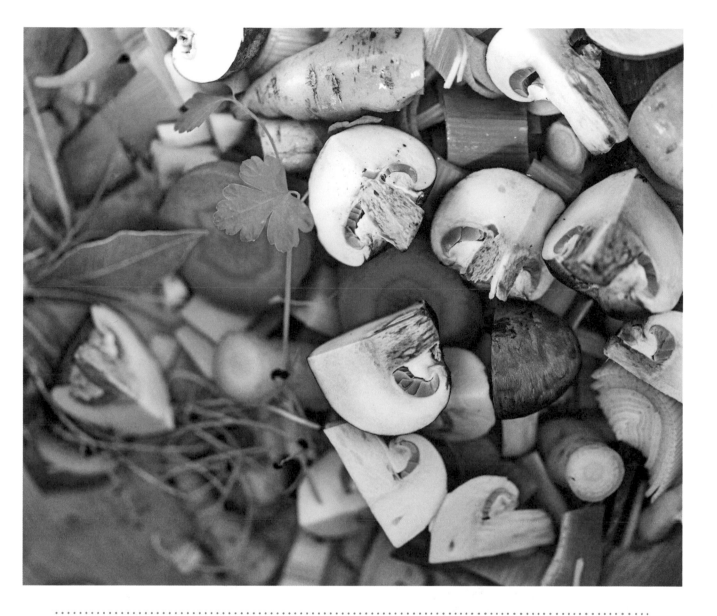

HOW TO CLEAN MUSHROOMS

It's tempting to clean the dirt from mushrooms with water, but that will make them soggy. Simply take a clean, dry kitchen towel or paper towel and gently rub the dirt from your mushrooms before preparing.

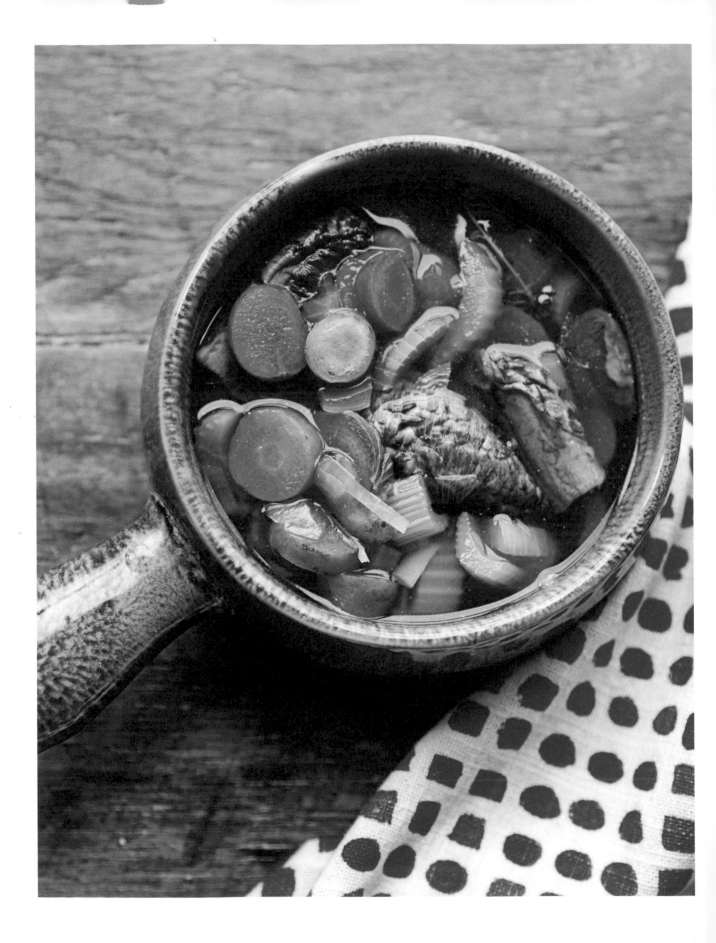

SAVORY MUSHROOM SOUP

 40 MINUTES   4   VEGAN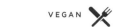

The mushroom broth and mushrooms in this soup provide a depth of taste and texture that rivals the "meatiest" of soups. The soup brings together the savory flavor of the mushrooms and the sweetness of cooked carrots and onions.

INGREDIENTS

1 tablespoon extra virgin olive oil

1 leek, sliced in ½ inch circles

1 medium yellow onion, diced

8 cups Mushroom Broth (recipe on page 92)

1 pound carrots, chopped

6 portobello mushrooms, sliced

2 cups celery, chopped

1 bay leaf

4 sprigs thyme, stems removed

DIRECTIONS

1. Add the **olive oil** to a deep pot over medium heat. Add the **leeks** and **onion** and sauté them for about 5 minutes.

2. Add the **broth** and **carrots** to the pot and bring the mixture to a low boil for 15 minutes.

3. Add the **remaining ingredients** and let the soup simmer for another 10 minutes.

BREAKFAST BARLEY "RISOTTO" WITH SAUTÉED MUSHROOMS, SHALLOTS, KALE, AND BOK CHOY

◑ 30 MINUTES   4 🍽   VEGAN 🍴

I have to admit, I was skeptical about savory oatmeal at first, but after trying a similar recipe from my French friend's mother, it got me thinking about the perfect breakfast food. Pearl barley, a firm grain, stands in for oats and cooks up like risotto. Sautéed with mushrooms, shallots, kale, and bok choy, this recipe becomes a surprisingly easy and delicious meal for breakfast, lunch, or dinner.

INGREDIENTS

1½ tablespoons extra virgin olive oil, divided

1 cup pearl barley

2 ½ cups Mushroom Broth (recipe on page 92)

3 scallions, thinly sliced, divided

1 tablespoon fresh ginger, peeled and grated

1 shallot, finely chopped

½ pound sliced mixed mushrooms

1 cup deveined and chopped curly kale

2 handfuls roughly chopped bok choy

1½ tablespoons tamari soy sauce

DIRECTIONS

1. Add ½ tablespoon of the **olive oil** to a deep pot or pressure cooker over low heat. Add the **barley** and sauté for 1 minute, being sure to stir the barley so that it doesn't burn.

2. Add the **Mushroom Broth** and half of the **scallions**. Simmer for 30 minutes without a pressure cooker. If you are using a pressure cooker, close the lid and cook the mixture for 20 minutes.

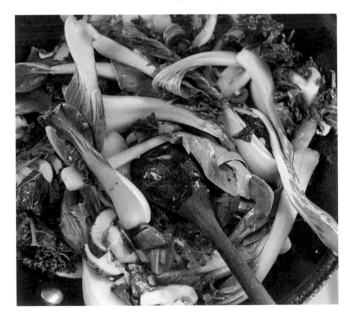

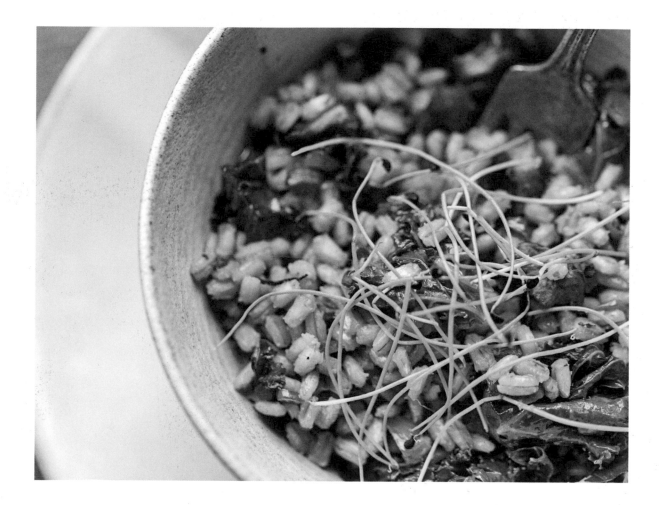

3. Heat the remaining 1 tablespoon of olive oil over medium heat in a nonstick skillet. Add the **ginger** and **shallot** and sauté them for 2 minutes or until they are fragrant.

4. Add the **mushrooms, kale, bok choy**, and 2 tablespoons of water to the skillet. Cover and sauté the mixture for 3–5 minutes until the kale and mushrooms become supple.

5. When the pearled barley is ready, drain any remaining liquid from pot, and add the mushroom mixture and **tamari sauce**. Stir. Serve the "risotto" in a bowl with the remaining scallions sprinkled on top.

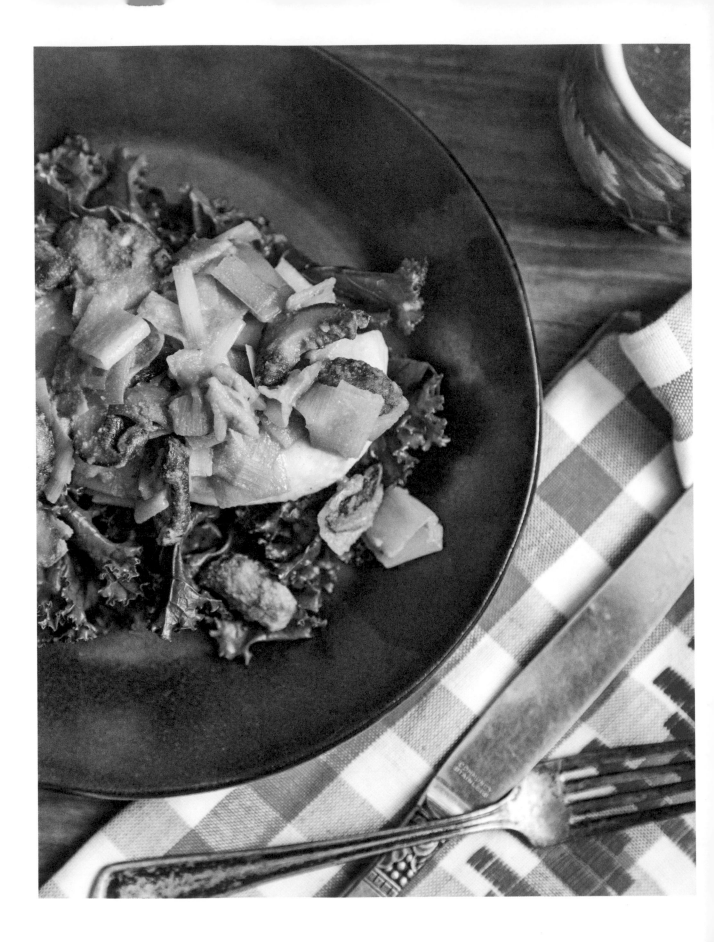

CHICKEN WITH SAUTÉED MUSHROOMS

🕐 25 MINUTES   2 🍽   NON-VEGETARIAN 🍴

Think of this dish as a lighter version of chicken Marsala. The sauce is less creamy, but not surprisingly, the mushrooms naturally give a robustness to the dish.

INGREDIENTS

1½ tablespoons of extra virgin olive oil, divided

2 whole organic chicken breasts

1 shallot

2 tablespoons ghee

⅓ cup leeks

1 cup mushrooms (I used the leftovers from Mushroom Broth

¼ cup Mushroom Broth (recipe on page 92)

1 teaspoon coconut flour

Pinch of sea salt, to taste

Pinch thyme

½ bunch kale, deveined and chopped

DIRECTIONS

1. Heat 1 tablespoon of the **olive oil** in a nonstick skillet over medium heat. Place the **chicken breasts** in the pan and sauté them evenly on both sides until they are fully cooked (about 10–12 minutes/side).

2. In a separate nonstick skillet, add the **ghee** and **leeks**. Cook for 4 minutes until the leeks are caramelized.

3. Add the **mushrooms** and a little **Mushroom Broth** to the skillet over low heat. Sprinkle the **coconut flour** over the mushrooms and stir thoroughly. Once the flour is absorbed, add the remainder of the Mushroom Broth, a sprinkle of **salt**, and some **thyme**. Cover and let the sauce thicken, stirring occasionally, for approximately 5 minutes. Remove the skillet and cover it.

4. Add the **kale**, the remaining ½ tablespoon of the olive oil, and some salt to the skillet. Sauté the kale for 3 minutes or until it wilts. Serve the chicken breasts over the kale and top with the mushroom sauce.

BRUSSELS SPROUTS AND MUSHROOM HASH WITH A SUNNY-SIDE UP EGG

🕐 25 MINUTES   2 🍽   VEGETARIAN 🌱

I love roasting Brussels sprouts, but sautéing them in a skillet with mushrooms gives them a whole new flavor, as they soak up the earthiness of their skillet counterparts. Toss on an egg, sunny-side up or poached, and you'll have a savory breakfast that won't spike your sugar.

INGREDIENTS

2 tablespoons extra virgin olive oil, divided

1 small shallot, minced

1 clove garlic, minced

1 portobello mushroom cap, chopped

1 pound Brussels sprouts, chopped

Salt, to taste

Juice of ½ lemon

2 large eggs

DIRECTIONS

1. Add 1 tablespoon of the **olive oil** and the **shallot** to a nonstick skillet over medium heat. Sauté for 2 minutes or until the shallot is translucent. Add the **garlic** and sauté for another minute.

2. Add the **mushrooms, Brussels sprouts**, and **salt** to the skillet. Cover the mixture and sauté for 5 minutes or until mushrooms and Brussels sprouts start to soften. Sprinkle with **lemon juice** halfway through and cover.

3. In a separate nonstick skillet, add the remaining 1 tablespoon of olive oil, then crack two **eggs** into the skillet. Cover the skillet and let the eggs steam for 2–3 minutes, making sure not to overcook the yolks. To serve, mound the Brussels sprout and mushroom hash onto two plates and place an egg on top of each.

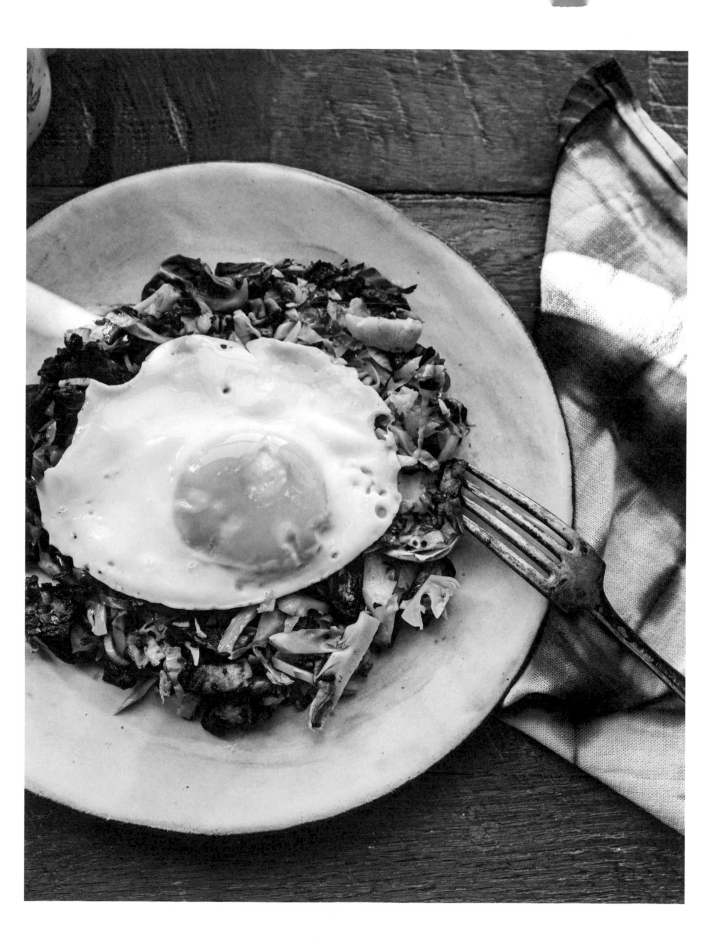

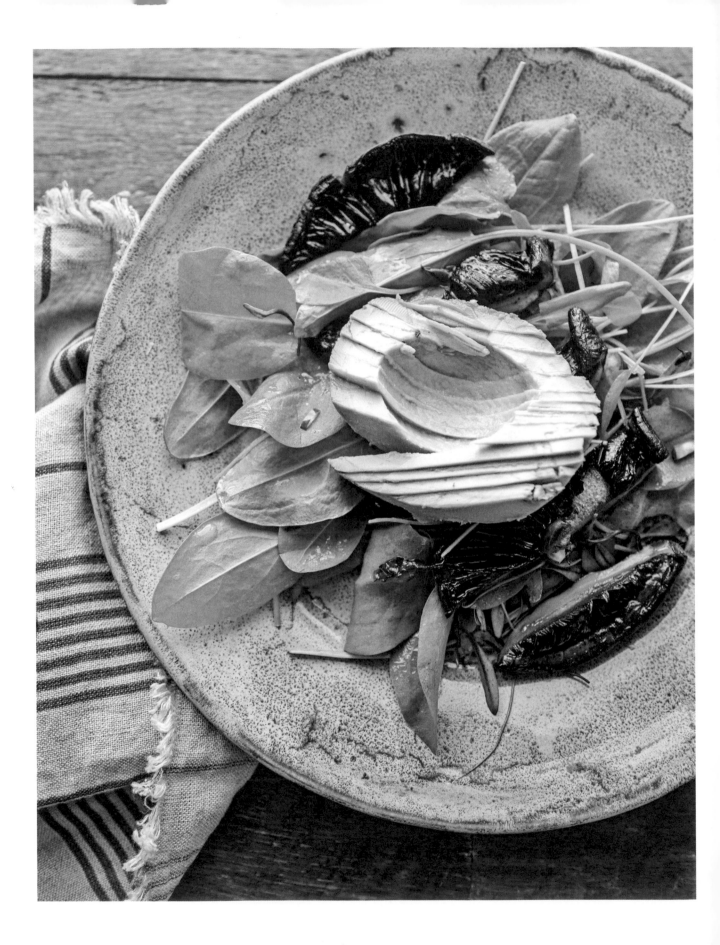

ROASTED BALSAMIC PORTOBELLO WITH GREENS AND AVOCADO

🕐 25 MINUTES   2 🍽   VEGAN ✗

Marinating and roasting portobello mushrooms releases their natural juices. In fact, if you've only eaten raw mushrooms, you may not believe how thick, meaty, and juicy they can actually be when they are cooked; even the most ardent meat lovers will be impressed with a roasted portobello, having to slice through the 'shroom with a sharp knife. It is, hands down, my favorite way of eating a 'bella. Add it to a freshly tossed salad topped with an avocado, and you have a power meal for any hour of the day.

INGREDIENTS

1 tablespoon extra virgin olive oil

2 portobello mushroom caps

1 tablespoon balsamic vinegar

Pinch of sea salt

Pinch of pepper

3 handfuls arugula or other salad greens, washed and dried

2 radishes, thinly sliced

Juice of ½ lemon

1 avocado, sliced in half, skin removed

DIRECTIONS

1. Preheat the oven to 400°F. Line a baking sheet with parchment paper. Brush the **olive oil** onto the **mushrooms**. Then brush them with the **balsamic vinegar**. Sprinkle the mushrooms with **salt** and **pepper**. Lay them on the baking sheet, gills down. Bake the mushrooms for 15 minutes.

2. While the mushrooms are baking, toss the **salad greens** with the **radishes** and **lemon juice**.

3. Remove the portobellos from the oven, place them on top of the salad, and top with half an **avocado**.

SCRAMBLED EGGS WITH KALE AND CREMINI MUSHROOMS

🕐 10 MINUTES　　2 🍽　　VEGETARIAN 🌿

The creminis you see in the store are actually just immature portobello mushrooms, but I find them much easier to work with than portobellos when I make an egg scramble. If you choose to use white button mushrooms, they work just as well—they're an even younger form of the cremini!

INGREDIENTS

2 tablespoons
extra virgin olive oil

1 shallot, thinly sliced

½ cup cremini
mushrooms, sliced

½ teaspoon sea salt

4 eggs, lightly beaten

Pinch of sea salt, to taste

Pinch of pepper, to taste

1 handful curly kale,
chopped

2 tablespoons scallion
microgreens (optional)

DIRECTIONS

1. Put 1 tablespoon of the **olive oil** and the sliced **shallot** into a nonstick skillet over medium heat. Sauté the shallot for 2 minutes or until it is translucent. Add the **mushrooms** and **salt** to the skillet and cook for another 3-4 minutes, or until the mushrooms are soft and golden brown around edges. Transfer the mushrooms to a plate.

2. Crack the **eggs** into a bowl, add salt and pepper to taste, and beat them until they are consistently blended. Add the remaining olive oil and eggs to the skillet. Cook the eggs over medium heat.

3. Before the eggs set, add the **kale** and let them steam for another 2 minutes. Use a spatula to break up and scramble the eggs. Transfer the eggs to a plate; spoon the mushrooms and shallots over the eggs; sprinkle the top with **scallion microgreens**, and serve.

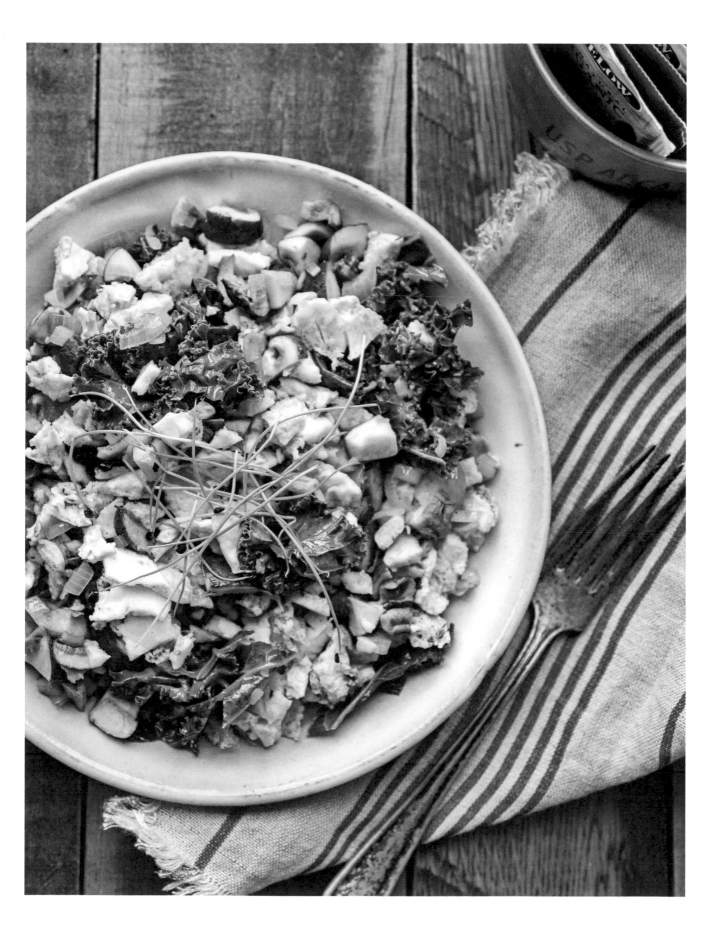

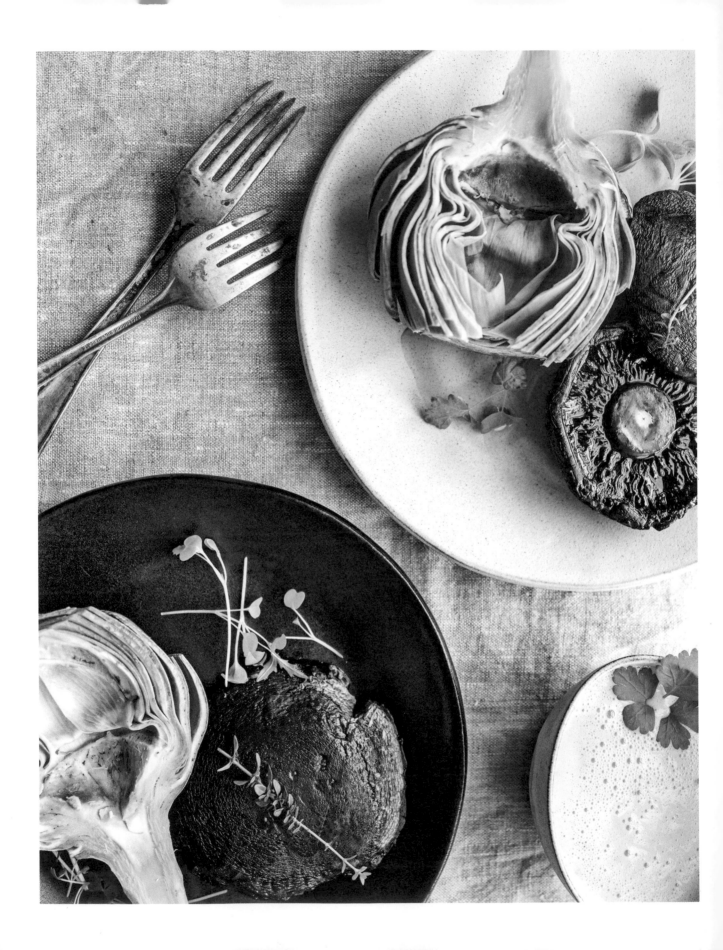

ROASTED PORTOBELLO MUSHROOMS WITH STEAMED ARTICHOKES AND AIOLI

🕐 25 MINUTES   2 🍽   VEGAN ✕

This is a special-occasion dish, largely because of the artichokes, members of the thistle family, which aren't always the easiest (or most practical) vegetable to prepare and eat. (Botanically, the artichoke is considered a flower.) However, I love artichokes and artichoke hearts, which you can find marinated in cans and jars. They're at the top of my snack list. These artichokes are more or less steamed and paired with juicy portobellos—a winning combination.

INGREDIENTS

Juice of 1 lemon

2 large artichokes

4 large portobello mushrooms

4 tablespoons extra virgin olive oil, divided

Pinch of sea salt, to taste

Pinch of pepper, to taste

2 shallots, finely sliced

2 cloves of garlic, minced

Aioli (see recipe on page 48)

DIRECTIONS

1. Put the **lemon juice** in a large mixing bowl, then fill three-quarters of the way with **water** and **ice**. Line a baking sheet with parchment paper.

2. Pare the **artichoke** heads to their hearts by cutting off the stems and breaking off leaves, all the way down to the choke. Remove the choke. Submerge the hearts in the iced lemon.

3. Place the **mushrooms** on the baking sheet and drizzle them with 2 tablespoons of the **olive oil**, **salt**, and **pepper**. Roast the mushrooms at 400°F for 15 minutes.

4. Heat the remaining 2 tablespoons of olive oil in a nonstick skillet and sauté the **shallots** over medium heat for 2 minutes or until the shallots are translucent. Add the **garlic** and a pinch of salt and pepper.

5. Thickly slice the artichoke hearts and add them to the skillet. Cook for 3-4 minutes, turning the mixture in the pan, and add just enough of the cold ice water you made in Step 1 to cover the mixture. Continue to cook it for 15 minutes, or until the water has evaporated and the artichokes are cooked through.

6. Plate the mushrooms and artichokes, and drizzle some **aioli** over the top. Serve.

MEAL MAP 4

HAVE **22** PANTRY STAPLES READY AND SHOP FOR THESE **16** MAIN INGREDIENTS TO MAKE **11** RECIPES AND **24** SERVINGS.

RECIPES

INGREDIENTS

3 red bell peppers

1 green pepper

3–4 red or green chile peppers

16 small to medium-size zucchini

2 medium-size yellow zucchini

1 cucumber

1½ pounds heirloom tomatoes

1 bunch Lacinato kale

1 bunch curly kale

8 ounces button mushrooms

3 15-ounce cans San Marzano tomatoes

1 7-ounce jar sun-dried tomatoes

2 teaspoons red chili paste

1 dozen pastured eggs

2 13.5-ounce cans coconut milk

3 pounds wild-caught shrimp

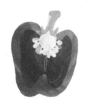

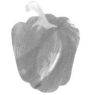

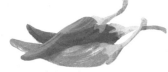

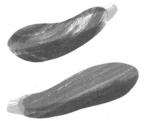

red ball peppers

green pepper

red or green chile peppers

zucchini

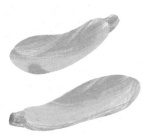

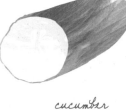

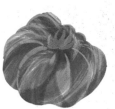

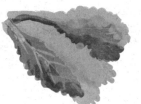

yellow zucchini

cucumber

heirloom tomatoes

Lacinato kale

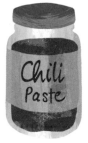

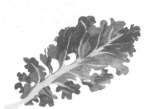

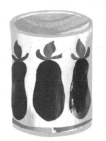

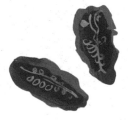

curly kale

button mushrooms

San Marzano tomatoes

sun-dried tomatoes

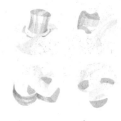

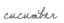

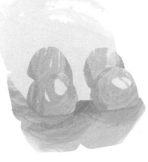

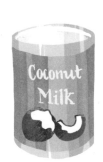

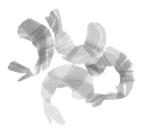

red chili paste

eggs

coconut milk

wild-caught shrimp

PANTRY STAPLES

Yellow onion × 3

Shallot × 2

Garlic × 2

Lemon × 3

Lime × 2

Quinoa

Pine nuts

Salt

Pepper

Extra virgin olive oil

Balsamic vinegar

Sherry vinegar

Paprika

Cumin

Coconut flour

Coconut oil

Basil

Mint

Parsley

Cilantro

Crushed red pepper

Vegetable broth

OPTIONAL

Watermelon

Microgreens

Goat's milk kefir

OPTIONAL SAUCES

Harissa

· ·

CHOOSING EGGS

Eggs can be confusing to buy because **free-range, cage-free**, **pastured**, and **organic** may not at all be what we envision when we think of each of those words. I'd say be sure to buy pastured, free-range eggs from a trusted local farmer. If you can visit the farm and see his or her chickens, even better! It's more likely that you'll be getting eggs from healthy chickens and therefore will get food rich in omega-3 fatty acids, which are important anti-inflammatory compounds that your body can't manufacture on its own. Commercially produced chickens are typically given very little space, pumped full of antibiotics, and fed processed, genetically modified grains. The food they eat gets converted into fat, fat stores quite a bit of pollutants, and this fat ends up in the yolks. So look for those healthier eggs from a farm that you trust.

· ·

SHAKSHUKA

◑ 30 MINUTES 2 🍽 VEGETARIAN 🌿

Popular in the Middle East, this dish, a poached egg nestled in a saucy bed of red peppers and tomatoes, is now common in many restaurants around the world, including the United States. The first time I had the authentic version of shakshuka was in Israel, where it is served with a side of sourdough bread—handy for sopping up the excess sauce. You can easily make this dish your own; just toss in some extra greens, like kale, chard, or spinach, or some broccoli florets for an added phytonutrient boost.

INGREDIENTS

2 tablespoons extra virgin olive oil

1 yellow onion, finely chopped

2 garlic cloves, finely chopped

1 red bell pepper, diced

1 teaspoon paprika

½ teaspoon cumin

1 cup zucchini, chopped

2 15-ounce cans San Marzano whole plum tomatoes

4 eggs

½ red or green chile pepper, or more to taste, minced

Pinch of sea salt, to taste

Pinch of pepper, to taste

½ cup washed, destemmed, and chopped Lacinato kale

1 large handful fresh basil

DIRECTIONS

1. Heat the **oil** in a nonstick skillet over medium heat. Add the **onion** and **garlic**, stirring them occasionally, until they are soft and golden brown, about 3 minutes.

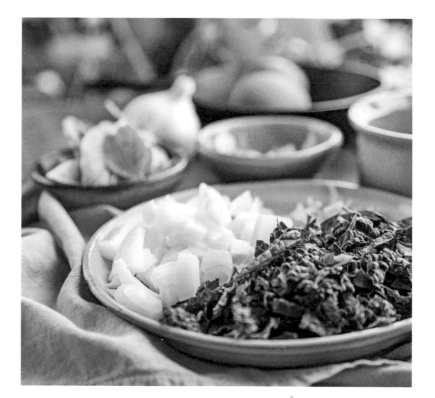

2. Add the **bell pepper**, **paprika**, and **cumin**, and cook for 2 minutes.

3. Meanwhile, transfer the **zucchini** and **tomatoes** to a blender and blend for about 2 minutes, or until the mixture is smooth. Pour the zucchini-tomato sauce mixture into the skillet and let it cook over low heat, covered, for 15 minutes.

4. While the skillet is still on the burner, make small divots in the sauce for the **eggs** and carefully crack the eggs into them. Add some **chiles**, **salt**, **pepper**, and the **kale**. Cover and cook over low heat for 5 more minutes, until the egg whites have set. Serve with some **fresh basil leaves**.

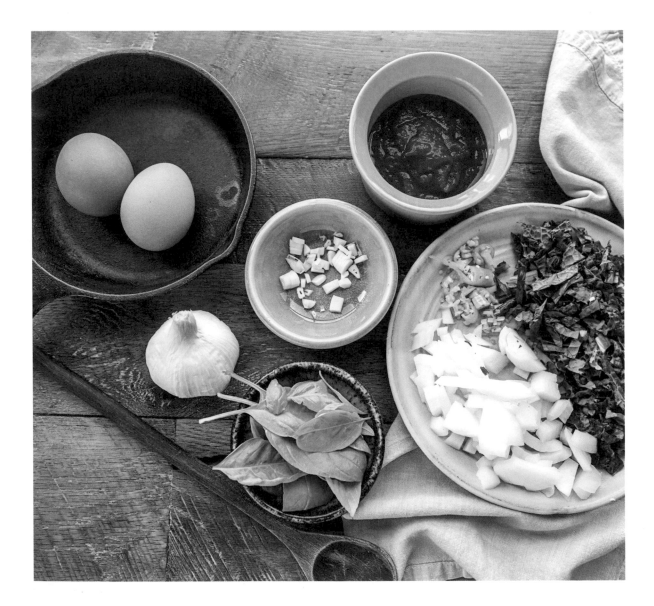

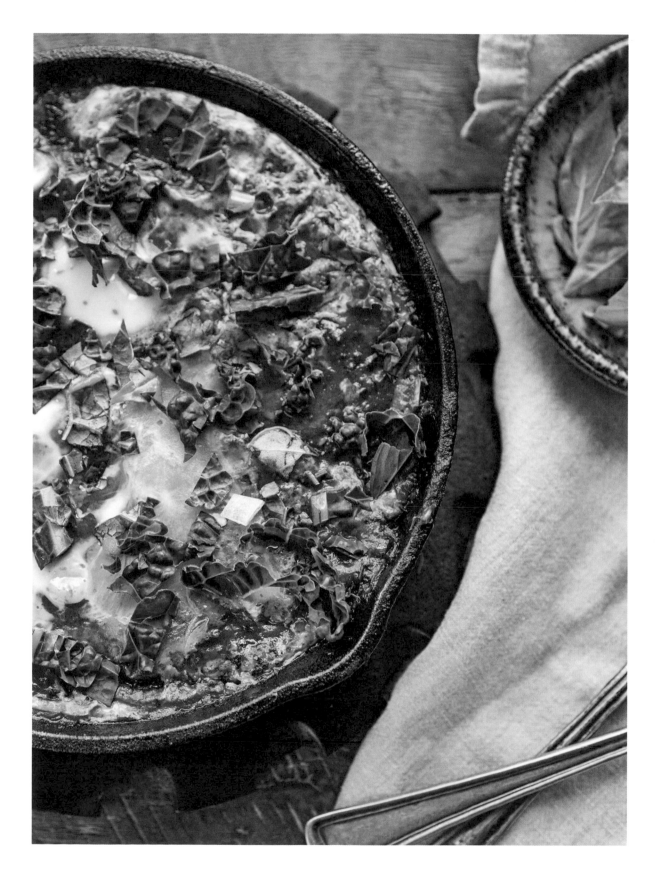

SPICY ZUCCHINI OMELET

🕐 10 MINUTES   2 🍽   VEGETARIAN 🌱

When I was growing up, we always had zucchini and eggs in the house, because my parents raised chickens for quite some time and zucchinis took over our garden every summer, up to the point that you'd begin to wonder if you could ever eat another zucchini again! (As I write this, I can hear my dad saying, "I can't even give these zucchinis away; there's just too many!") Combining zucchini and eggs with some green or red chiles and fresh basil will pique your taste buds, even if you're tired of green squash!

INGREDIENTS

2 tablespoons extra virgin olive oil, divided

1 shallot, finely diced

1 cup zucchini, chopped finely and patted dry

5 eggs

2 green or red chiles, seeds removed, cut finely

1 teaspoon cumin

6 basil leaves, chopped

Harissa or sugar-free hot sauce (optional)

DIRECTIONS

1. Add 1 tablespoon of the **olive oil** to a nonstick skillet over medium heat. Cook the **shallot** and **zucchini** for about 5 minutes until the mixture is golden, stirring after a couple of minutes so that it will cook evenly. Remove half of the mixture from the pan.

2. Whisk the **eggs** with half the **chiles** and the **cumin**. Add half the mixture to the pan and make sure the base of the pan is coated evenly. Cover and cook for about 2 minutes over medium heat until the eggs have firmed up.

3. Add one quarter of the **basil leaves** to the omelet and fold it in half. Sprinkle half of the remaining chiles and basil on top. If more heat is desired, add a little **harissa** or **hot sauce**.

4. Repeat the steps to make the second omelet.

* Shown with sautéed sweet potato.

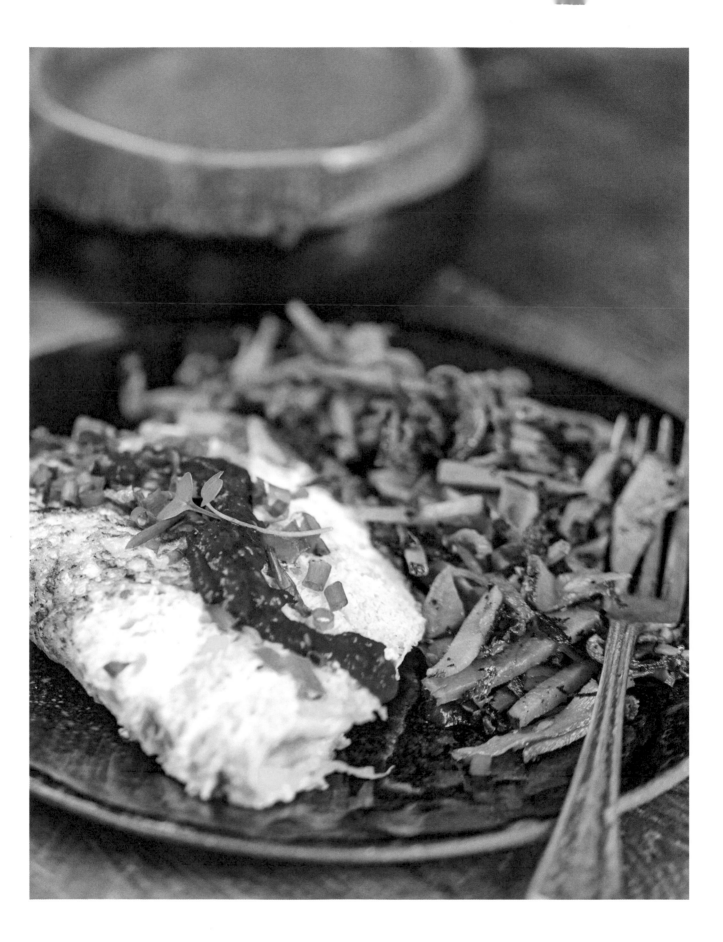

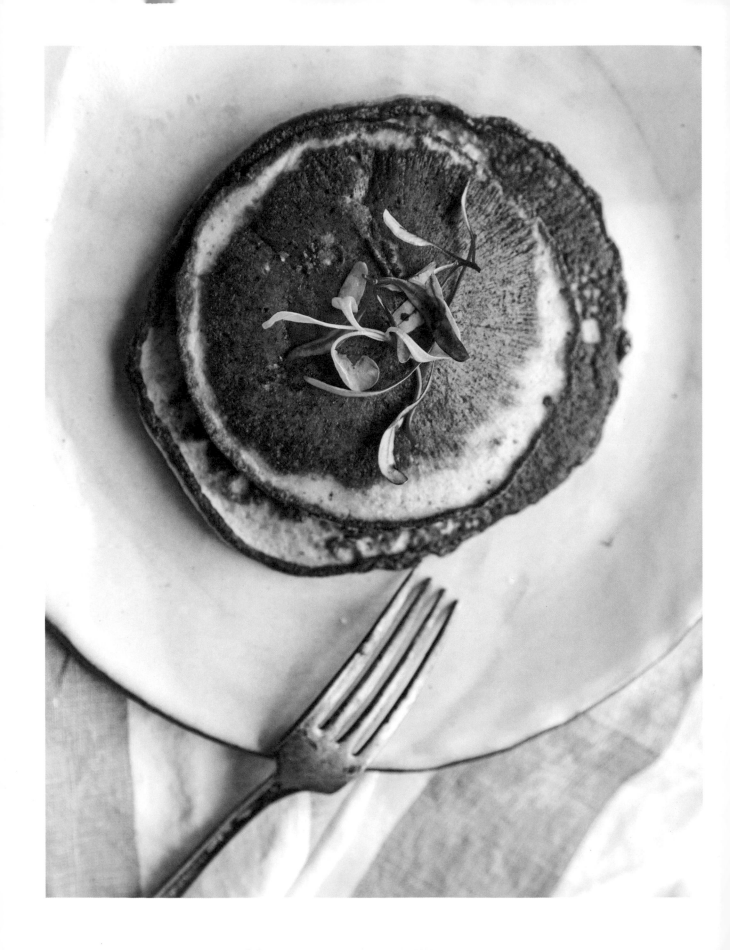

ZUCCHINI PANCAKES

🕐 15 MINUTES   2 🍽   VEGETARIAN 🌱

When I was growing up, my mother used to cook her father's recipe for pancakes for me, my brother, and his friend, Peter. Pancake-eating competitions ensued (I'd always lose), and sometimes my brother and Peter would scarf down as many as 20 or 30 pancakes apiece. I wouldn't suggest going that far overboard, but this recipe, which is loosely based on my grandfather's recipe, will definitely turn you into a flapjack lover. For a creamy, tangy alternative to maple syrup, use a little goat's milk kefir.

INGREDIENTS

1½ cups shredded zucchini

3 eggs

3 tablespoons coconut flour

1 clove garlic, diced

¼ teaspoon sea salt

⅛ teaspoon pepper

1 tablespoon coconut oil, plus more as needed

1 cup goat's milk kefir (optional)

DIRECTIONS

1. Blend the **zucchini**, **eggs**, **flour**, **garlic**, **salt**, and **pepper** in a blender to form a pancake batter.

2. In a nonstick skillet, melt the **coconut oil** over medium heat and pour about 2 tablespoons of mixture into the skillet. Fry the first side until it starts to bubble around the edges, approximately 2–3 minutes. Flip and fry on the other side until golden brown. Repeat for the remaining pancakes, adding more coconut oil to the skillet if necessary. Top with **kefir**, if you have it.

ZUCCHINI NOODLES WITH SUN-DRIED TOMATO AND BASIL

🕐 15 MINUTES   2 🍽   VEGAN 🍴

The easiest way to turn zucchini into noodles is to use a spiralizer, and even though the zucchini tastes no different than if you chopped or diced it, you do experience the food differently—it's more like eating a fresh, crisp summer pasta than just a veggie.

INGREDIENTS

1 small green zucchini

1 small yellow zucchini

Juice of 1 lemon

¼ teaspoon crushed red pepper flakes

¼ cup sun-dried tomatoes

Pinch of pepper, to taste

¼ cup fresh basil, chopped

2 ounces microgreens (optional)

DIRECTIONS

1. Spiralize the **zucchini**.

2. Add the **lemon juice** and **crushed red pepper flakes** to the zucchini noodles. Top with the **sun-dried tomatoes**, **pepper**, and **basil**. Sprinkle with **microgreens**, if you have them.

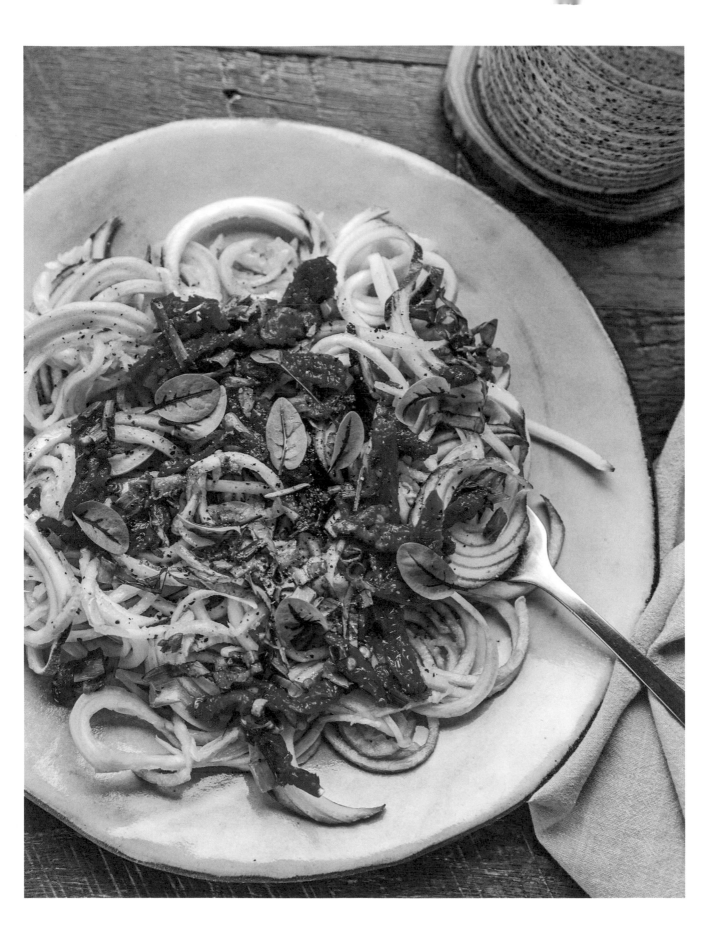

ZUCCHINI CARPACCIO WITH SUN-DRIED TOMATO, PARSLEY, MINT, AND BASIL

⏲ 10 MINUTES   2 🍽   VEGAN 🍴

This is my go-to potluck dish for summer and fall parties. Thinly slice small zucchinis and arrange them on a serving platter. The presentation alone will wow your guests.

INGREDIENTS

2 tablespoons pine nuts

¼ cup sun-dried tomatoes

¼ cup extra virgin olive oil, divided

1 juice of lemon

8 small zucchini, thinly sliced

Zest of 1 lemon

1 tablespoon basil chiffonade

1 tablespoon mint chiffonade

1 tablespoon parsley roughly chopped

⅛ teaspoon pepper

¼ teaspoon crushed red pepper (optional)

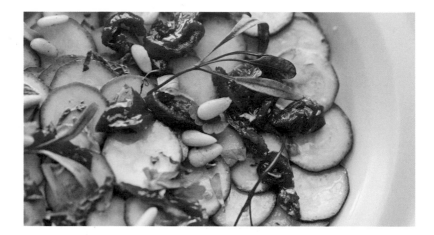

DIRECTIONS

1. Toast the **pine nuts** for 1 minute in a nonstick skillet over low heat with 1 tablespoon of the **olive oil**. Remove the pine nuts. Next sauté the **sun-dried tomatoes** over medium heat for 2 minutes. Set the skillet aside.

2. Mix together the **lemon juice** and the remainder of the olive oil in a small bowl. Add the sliced **zucchini** to the bowl and toss.

3. Arrange the zucchini on individual plates, top with the sun-dried tomatoes, and drizzle with any remaining olive oil and lemon juice. Scatter the pine nuts over the top.

4. Sprinkle the **lemon zest**, **basil**, **mint**, and **parsley** over the top. Add **pepper** and a dash of **crushed red pepper** as optional seasoning.

GRILLED PEPPERS, ZUCCHINI, MUSHROOMS, AND SHRIMP WITH BALSAMIC VINEGAR

🕐 20 MINUTES   4 🍽   PESCATARIAN 🐟

This is my dad's specialty dish, and let me tell you, he feels proud whenever he makes it, largely because he gets the fresh zucchini and some of the peppers straight from his garden. I even went back home to Pennsylvania to photograph this dish because I couldn't imagine making it without my dad!

INGREDIENTS

2 tablespoons extra virgin olive oil

¼ cup balsamic vinegar

Pinch of sea salt, to taste

Pinch of pepper, to taste

1 yellow onion, chopped

1 green zucchini, sliced

1 yellow zucchini, sliced

½ red pepper, chopped

½ green pepper, chopped

8 ounces button mushrooms, quartered

1 pound fresh shrimp, cleaned and deveined

DIRECTIONS

1. Combine the **olive oil**, **vinegar**, **salt**, and **pepper** in a shallow dish. Marinate the **onion**, **green zucchini**, **yellow zucchini**, **red pepper**, **green pepper**, and **mushrooms** in the mixture for 10 minutes or more.

2. Add the marinated vegetables and the **shrimp** to a grill basket. Grill over a medium flame, stirring frequently, for about 5 minutes. Make sure the shrimp turns pink and cooks thoroughly. Plate and serve.

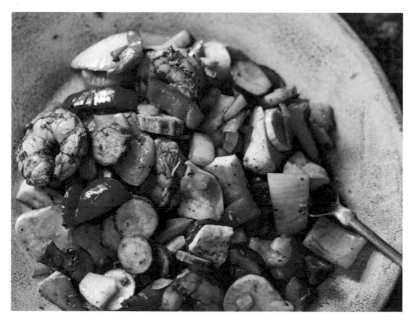

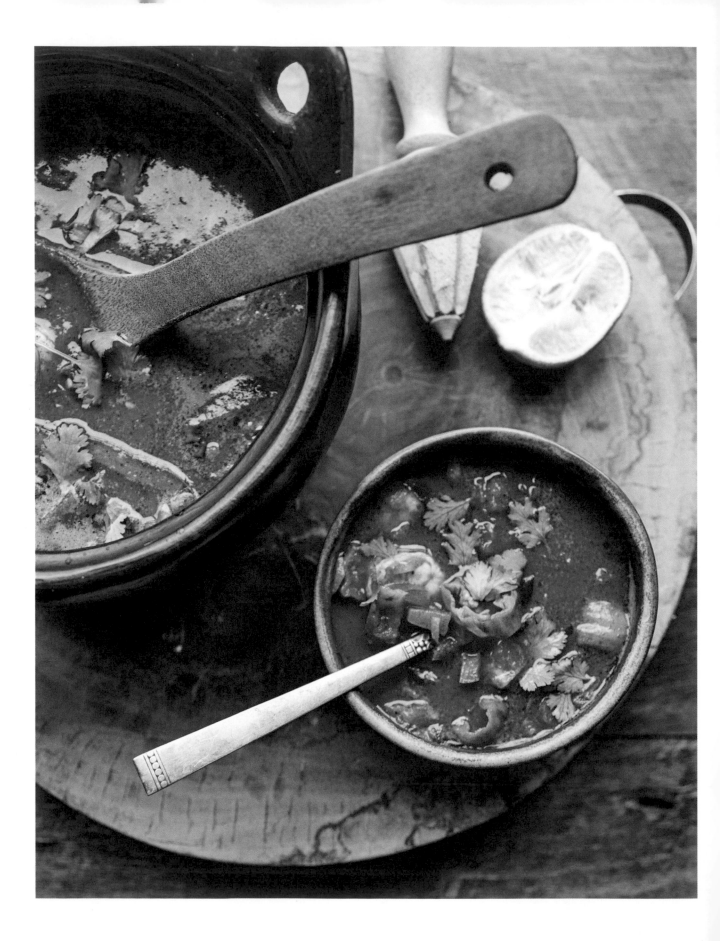

BRAZILIAN SHRIMP SOUP
(*MOQUECA DE CAMARÃO*)

🕐 **45** MINUTES   **2** 🍽   PESCATARIAN 🐟

Thanks to a Brazilian former roommate, I got a taste of some of the dishes from her homeland. This Brazilian shrimp soup, known as *moqueca de camarão* in Portuguese, was one of my favorites. The shrimp are simmered in a robust, full-flavored broth that includes red and green bell peppers, tomatoes, and coconut milk. The red bell pepper, a mature version of green bell peppers, is a powerhouse of flavor and nutrients, and its vitamins C, A, B$_6$, and E, along with folate and fiber, is off the charts.

INGREDIENTS

2 tablespoons extra virgin olive oil

1 yellow onion, diced

½ red bell pepper

½ green bell pepper

4 garlic cloves, diced

1 red or green chile pepper

¼ teaspoon sea salt

1 15-ounce can San Marzano tomatoes

1 13.5-ounce can coconut milk

2 pounds shrimp, cleaned and deveined

⅛ teaspoon black pepper

Juice of 1 lime

4 cups water

½ cup parsley

¼ cup cilantro

DIRECTIONS

1. In a deep pot heat the **olive oil** over low heat. Add the **onion, red pepper, green pepper,** and **garlic** and cook stirring occasionally until the onion and pepper are soft, about 5 minutes.

2. Add the **chile, salt, tomatoes,** and **coconut milk** to the pot. Bring the broth to a simmer and then stir in the **shrimp**. Simmer, stirring occasionally, until the shrimp are just done, 3–5 minutes. Stir in the **black pepper, lime juice, water, parsley,** and **cilantro.** Simmer for another minute. Scoop into bowls and serve.

GAZPACHO

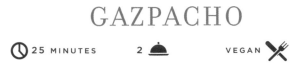

25 MINUTES   2   VEGAN

When tomatoes are in season, gazpacho becomes my go-to soup. It's easy to make, naturally sweet, and so refreshing—and it's an excellent meal or snack. Make a batch of gazpacho and pack it in a mason jar to sip throughout the day or have as a meal. If you like your soups chunky, dice some cucumbers, peppers, and tomatoes and toss them on top of the puree. Or, if you like your gazpacho extra smooth, strain the puree through a cheesecloth or nut milk bag.

INGREDIENTS

2 garlic cloves, minced

1 red bell pepper, seeds removed and sliced

1 pound heirloom tomatoes, peeled, cut, and seeded

Pinch of sea salt, to taste

Pinch of pepper, to taste

1 large cucumber, sliced

½ small shallot

2 tablespoons sherry vinegar

3 tablespoons extra virgin olive oil, divided

2 cups watermelon cubes (optional)

1 tablespoon chopped fresh basil (optional)

2 ounces microgreens (optional)

DIRECTIONS

1. Add the **garlic**, **red pepper**, **tomatoes**, **salt**, **pepper**, **cucumber**, **shallot**, **vinegar**, and 2 tablespoons of the **olive oil** to a blender. Blend the mixture on high for 2 minutes. If you have some fresh **watermelon**, toss it in as well and blend for another minute.

2. Chill the soup for 20 minutes, pour it into bowls, drizzle with the remaining olive oil, and top with **fresh basil** and **microgreens**.

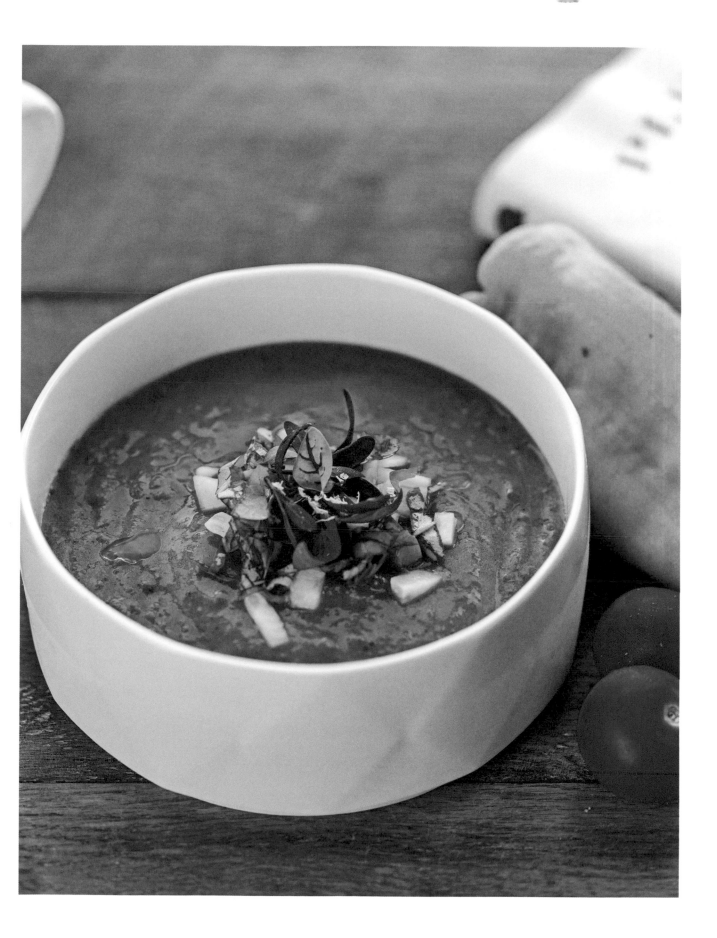

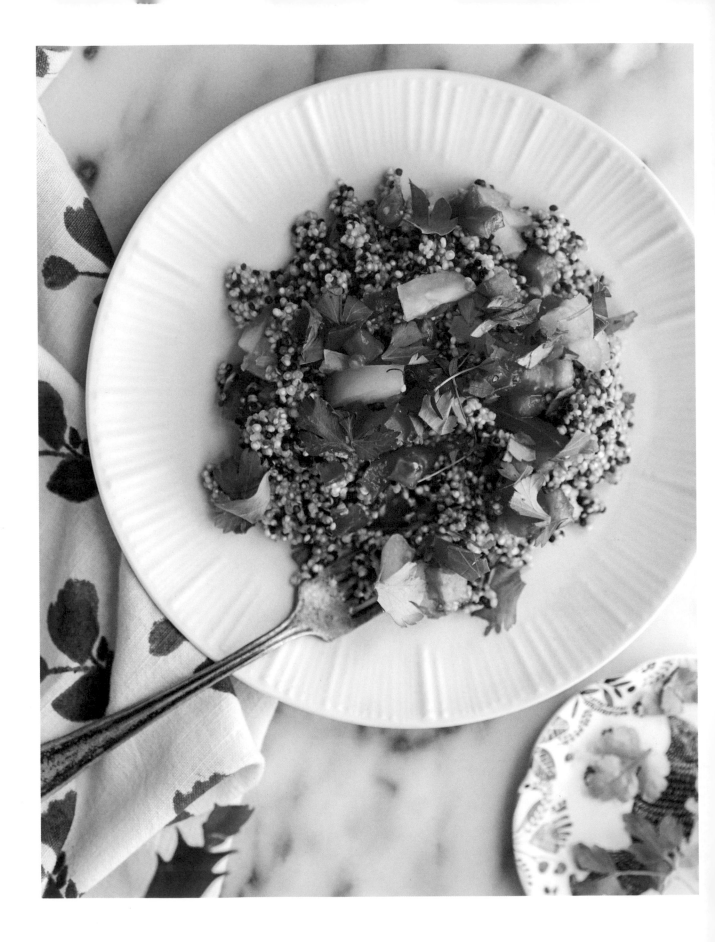

QUINOA WITH HEIRLOOM TOMATO AND PARSLEY

🕐 20 MINUTES   2 🍽   VEGAN ✗

Quinoa is an ancient grain that originated in Peru and Bolivia, and it has become popular—or, should I say, trendy. This is not without good reason: Quinoa is a complete protein, since it contains all of the essential amino acids that your body needs, in addition to two others—tryptophan and valine. Quinoa is considered a pseudograin because it's not really classified as a cereal grain, but it's cooked, prepared, and eaten like one. Quinoa is closely related to more familiar edibles, including beets, chard, and spinach. For vegetarians and vegans who are looking to get more protein into their diet, quinoa is a great choice.

INGREDIENTS

½ cup quinoa

1 cup vegetable broth, store-bought, or use the recipe for Homemade Vegetable Broth on page 66

1 medium heirloom tomato, diced

2 tablespoons parsley, diced

Pinch of sea salt, to taste

DIRECTIONS

1. Bring the **quinoa** and **broth** to a boil in a medium saucepan. Reduce the heat to low, cover the saucepan, and let the broth simmer until the quinoa is tender and most of the liquid has been absorbed, about 15 minutes. Fluff the quinoa with a fork and let it cool.

2. Top the quinoa with the **tomato** and **parsley**. Sprinkle it with some **salt** and serve.

BREAKFAST QUINOA WITH SUN-DRIED TOMATO AND SHREDDED ZUCCHINI

🕐 20 MINUTES　　　2 🍽　　　VEGAN 🍴

Sun-dried tomatoes have a concentrated flavor, and since quinoa and zucchini are both mild tasting, the tomatoes definitely take center stage in this dish.

INGREDIENTS

½ cup quinoa

1 cup vegetable broth, store-bought, or use the recipe for Homemade Vegetable Broth on page 66

¼ cup sun-dried tomatoes

1 cup shredded zucchini

DIRECTIONS

1. Bring the **quinoa** and **broth** to a boil in a medium saucepan. Reduce the heat to low, cover the saucepan, and let the broth simmer until the quinoa is tender and most of the liquid has been absorbed, about 15 minutes. Fluff the quinoa with a fork and let it cool.

2. While the quinoa is cooking, heat a nonstick skillet over low heat and sauté the **sun-dried tomatoes** and **zucchini** for 2 minutes, stirring.

3. Plate the quinoa and top with the sun-dried tomato and zucchini mix. Serve.

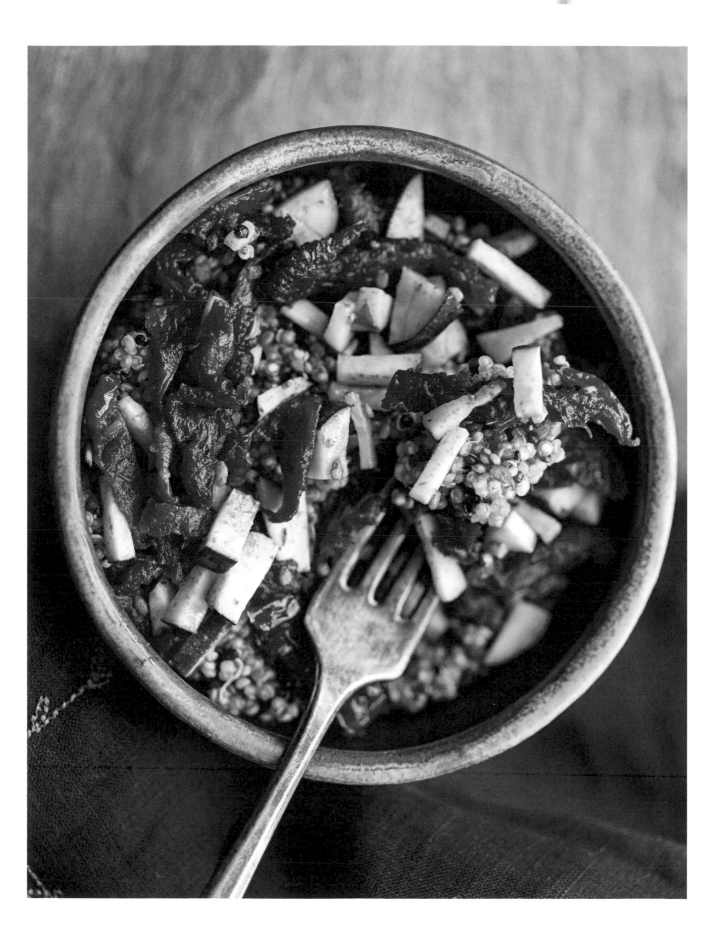

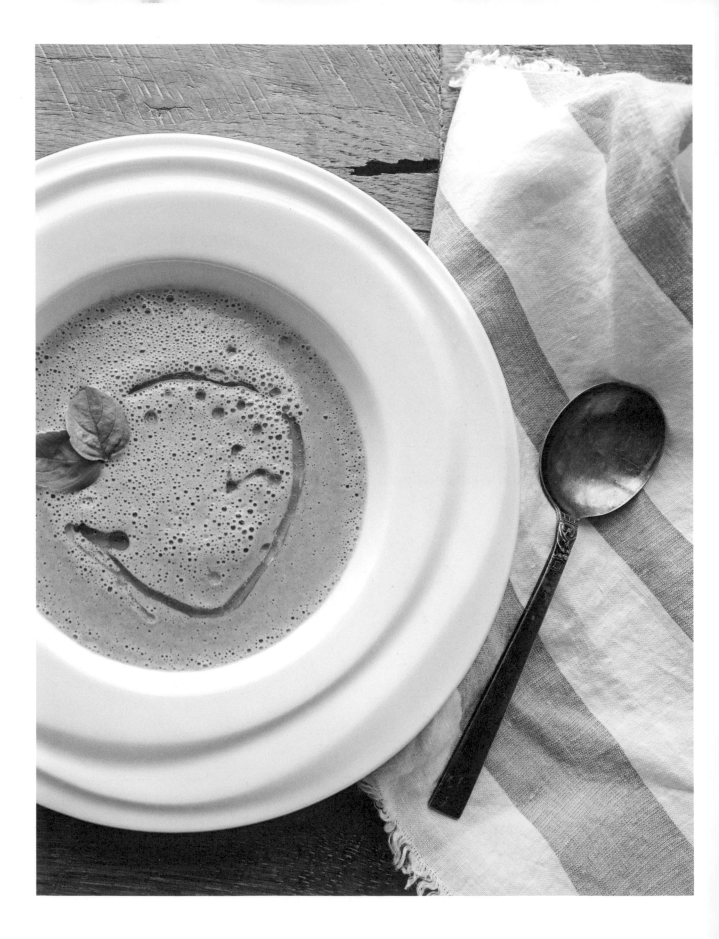

SPICY ZUCCHINI SOUP

🕐 10 MINUTES   2 🍽   VEGAN ✕

My mother would often make zucchini bread or fried zucchini, but it wasn't until I had it raw and lightly sautéed that I really began to appreciate zucchini for what it is. At the height of its growing season, you do begin to wonder if you can possibly eat any more of it—and try to peddle it to neighbors, coworkers, and the guy at the gas station—but pureeing it with a handful of kale, coconut milk, and chiles gives you a new and exciting way to eat zucchini. You can freeze this soup as well, so that once zucchini season has passed you can thaw, simmer, and serve it warm.

INGREDIENTS

2 tablespoons coconut oil

2 medium zucchini, diced

2 cups vegetable broth, store-bought, or use the recipe for Homemade Vegetable Broth on page 66

1 cup curly kale

¼ cup fresh mint

1-2 teaspoons red chili paste

½ can (6.75 ounces) coconut milk

Juice of 1 lime

1 tablespoon extra virgin olive oil

¼ teaspoon sea salt (optional)

DIRECTIONS

1. Heat the **coconut oil** in a medium saucepan. Add the **zucchini** and sauté for 2 minutes. Add the **vegetable broth** and simmer over medium heat for 4–6 minutes.

2. Add the **kale, mint,** and **chili paste**. Cover the saucepan and cook the broth for 2 minutes, then blend the mixture with an immersion blender or regular blender until it's green and creamy.

3. Add the **coconut milk** to the soup, blend it some more, add the **lime juice,** and taste. Add **salt,** if necessary. Top the soup with a little swirl of **olive oil** and serve.

MEAL MAP 5

Have **21** pantry staples ready and shop for these **17** main ingredients to make **11** recipes and **28** servings.

RECIPES

INGREDIENTS

2 sweet potatoes

6 green zucchini

1 yellow zucchini

1 bunch asparagus

4 cups English peas

2 dozen snow peas

6 ounces microgreen mix

3 medium Yukon gold potatoes

6 bunches kale

6 cups baby kale

1 bunch carrots

1 green chile pepper

1 small red cabbage

8 cherry tomatoes

4 ounces bacon, dry cured, dry rubbed, or uncured

8 pastured eggs

2 sole fillets

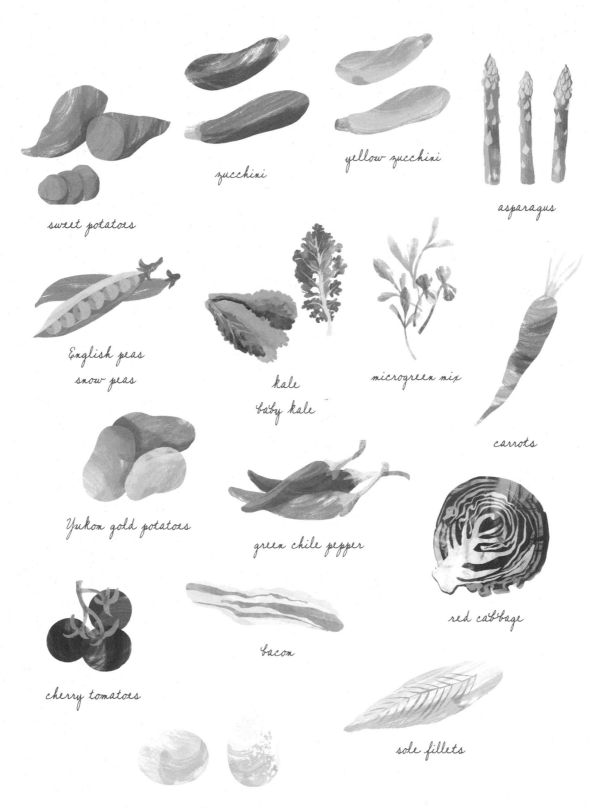

zucchini

yellow zucchini

asparagus

sweet potatoes

English peas
snow peas

kale
baby kale

microgreen mix

carrots

Yukon gold potatoes

green chile pepper

red cabbage

cherry tomatoes

bacon

sole fillets

eggs

PANTRY STAPLES

Shallots × 6

Garlic × 1

Yellow onion × 1

Lemons × 4

Walnuts

Salt

Pepper

Extra virgin olive oil

Ghee

Crushed red pepper

Cumin

Paprika

Vegetable or chicken broth

Distilled vinegar

Apple cider vinegar

Cilantro

Basil

Parsley

Mint

Thyme

Nutritional yeast

SUNNY-SIDE UP EGGS WITH SWEET POTATO AND ZUCCHINI HASH

🕐 **15** MINUTES   **2** 🍽   VEGETARIAN 🌿

Even though zucchini are creamy and firm, they have a high water content (around 95 percent), which means they don't crisp up as easily as sweet potatoes (their water content is around 77 percent). Sweet potatoes, despite their name, are not a potato at all, but, rather, a root vegetable in the morning glory family. There are many different varieties of sweet potatoes, and the general rule of thumb is the darker the variety, the higher the carotene content, which is good for your skin and eyes. And although the sweet potato is starchy, it has been shown to stabilize blood sugar levels and sensitize insulin, likely due to the fiber content, which is why I like to leave the skin on!

INGREDIENTS

2 tablespoons extra virgin olive oil, divided

1 sweet potato, julienned

1 zucchini, julienned

2 eggs

Pinch of sea salt, to taste

Pinch of pepper, to taste

DIRECTIONS

1. Add 1 tablespoon of the **olive oil** to a nonstick skillet. Add the **sweet potato** and sauté for 8 minutes or until it starts to soften. Move the sweet potato to one side of the pan and add the **zucchini**. Sauté the zucchini for 2 minutes. Remove the sweet potato/zucchini mixture from the skillet.

2. Add the remaining 1 tablespoon of olive oil to the skillet. Crack the **eggs** into the skillet. Cover the skillet and let the eggs steam over medium heat for about 1 minute, or until the whites of the eggs are opaque and the yolks have set on the outside. Sprinkle the eggs with a little **salt** and **pepper**. Use a metal spatula to carefully remove the eggs from the skillet, being careful not to puncture the yolks.

3. Divide the sweet potato and zucchini hash between two plates and place an egg on top of each.

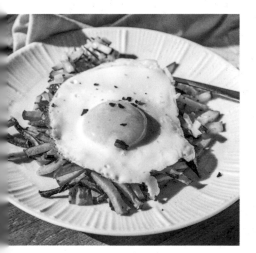

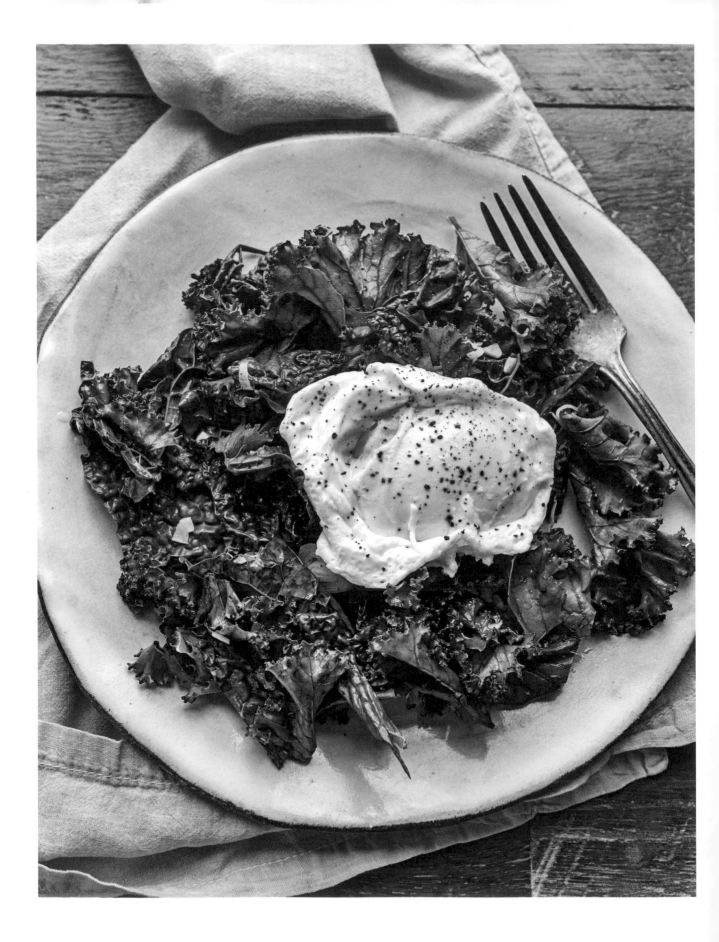

POACHED EGGS WITH SPICED KALE

🕐 **15** MINUTES   **2** 🍽   VEGETARIAN 🌿

Talk about a power breakfast! One quality, pasture-fed, farm-fresh egg will give you at least 6 grams of protein, and the kale will give you around 2–3 grams per cup, which is about one sixth of what a typical woman needs and one seventh of what is suggested for men per day. Not to mention that the eggs, kale, and alliums, like shallots and garlic, in this recipe are rich sources of sulfur-containing proteins and compounds, which are essential to the health of your body's tissues and membranes.

INGREDIENTS

2 eggs

2 tablespoons distilled vinegar

2 tablespoons ghee

2 shallots, finely diced

2 garlic cloves, minced

1 bunch kale, washed, destemmed, and roughly chopped

½ cup vegetable broth, store-bought, or use the recipe for Homemade Vegetable Broth on page 66

¼ teaspoon sea salt

⅛ teaspoon pepper

¼ teaspoon paprika

Juice of 1 lemon

Crushed red pepper flakes, to taste (optional)

DIRECTIONS

1. Poach **1 egg** in water with the **distilled vinegar** in medium saucepan for 4 minutes. Remove the egg with a slotted spoon and place it on a paper towel on a plate. Do the same for the second egg, using the same water.

2. Melt the **ghee** in a nonstick skillet over medium-high heat. Add the **shallots** and sauté, stirring, for 2 minutes or until they are translucent. Add the **garlic** and sauté for another minute or until the garlic is fragrant. Add the **kale** and sauté for 2 minutes or until it begins to wilt. Add the **broth, salt, pepper, paprika,** and **lemon juice**. Simmer for another 3 minutes.

3. To serve, divide the kale between two plates and add an egg to each. Sprinkle with **crushed red pepper flakes** and enjoy.

SAUTÉED KALE WITH BACON-EGG SCRAMBLE

🕐 10 MINUTES   4 🍽   NON-VEGETARIAN 🍴🍽

Add a slice of bacon or two to a dish of high-protein kale and eggs, and you get a bonus of 6 more grams of protein. I don't cook with bacon often and offer just a couple of recipes in this book that include it, so I'd love for you to consider it a luxury—something crispy, salty, juicy, and luscious all wrapped into one that can be enjoyed once in a while, not every day. You'll find how much more you appreciate bacon when you eat less of it!

INGREDIENTS

4 strips bacon

4 eggs

1 handful kale, stems removed and roughly chopped

Pinch of crushed red pepper flakes, to taste

DIRECTIONS

1. Sauté the **bacon slices** in a nonstick skillet over medium heat for 5 minutes (or until desired crispness), turning the bacon after 2–3 minutes to make sure it is evenly cooked. Transfer the bacon to a paper towel to soak up any excess grease. Leave the bacon grease in the skillet.

2. Crack the **eggs** into a small bowl, whisk them thoroughly, and then pour them into the skillet. Add the **kale** to the skillet and let it steam for 2 minutes. Using a spatula, break up the eggs to scramble them. Reduce the heat and cook the egg and kale mixture for another minute. Sprinkle on some **red pepper flakes** and serve.

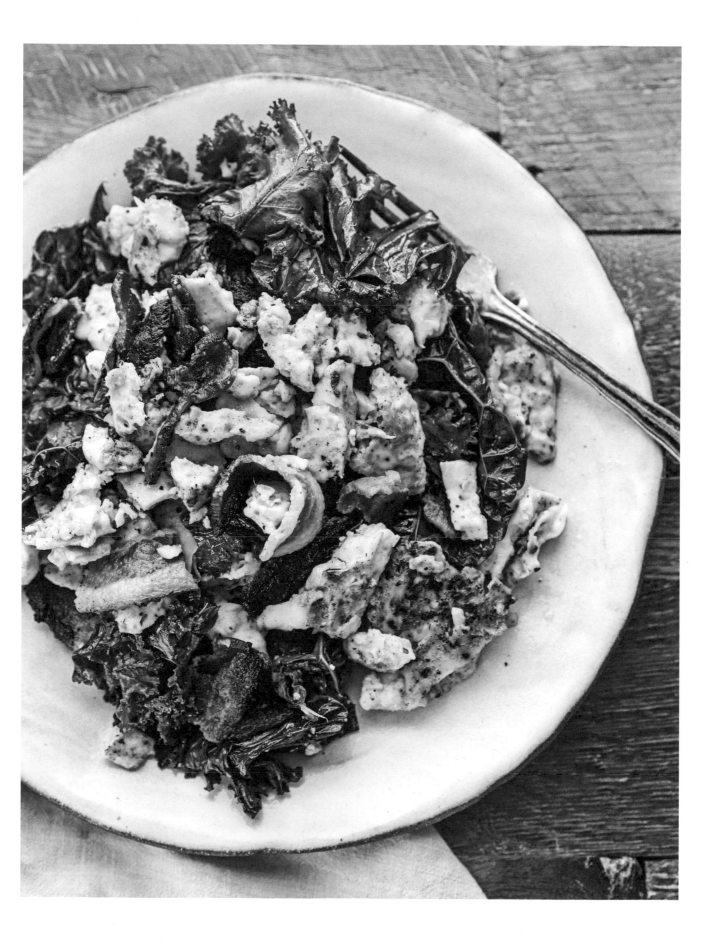

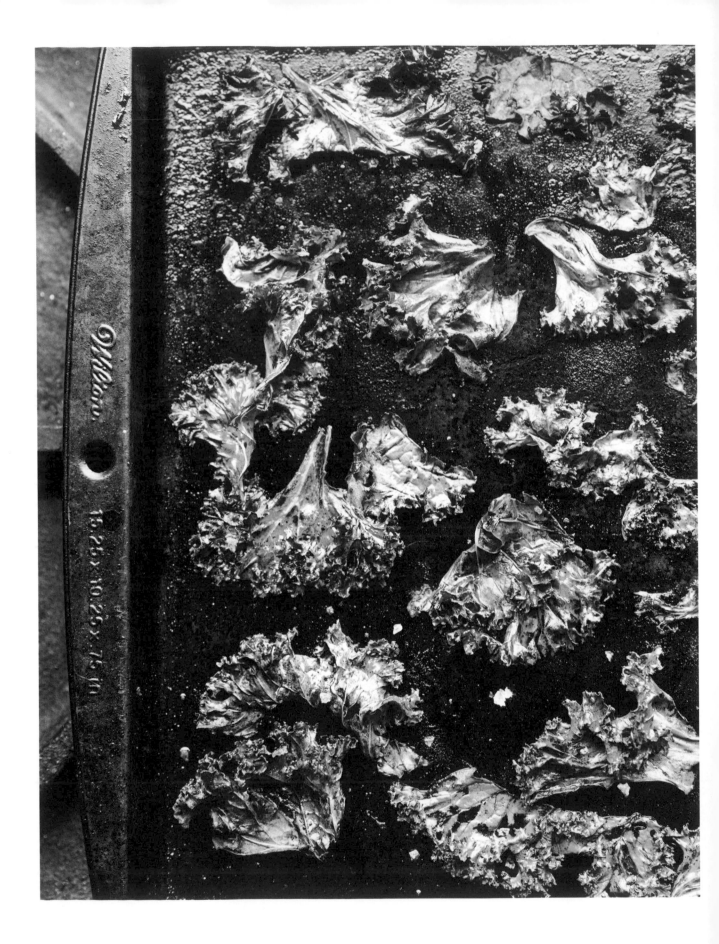

LEMON KALE CHIPS

🕐 10 MINUTES   2 🍽   VEGAN ✕

I have yet to find a kid or an adult who doesn't like a kale chip. Sure, it sounds unappetizing—almost "too healthy" to be good, but the crunchiness and just-enough-saltiness of kale chips is satisfying and much healthier for you than potato chips. Baking kale doesn't diminish the vitamin content at all, which means you're getting a substantial dose of vitamins K, A, C, and B_6 as well as other important minerals each time you enjoy these chips. Just go easy on the oil and salt to preserve their status as a healthy chip.

INGREDIENTS

1 bunch kale, roughly chopped

2 tablespoons extra virgin olive oil

2 tablespoons lemon juice

¼ teaspoon sea salt

¼ teaspoon cumin

DIRECTIONS

1. Place the chopped **kale** in a large bowl. With your hands, massage the **olive oil**, **lemon juice**, and **salt** into the kale until it's supple.

2. Place the kale on a parchment-lined baking sheet. Sprinkle the kale with the **cumin**. Bake the kale at 350°F for 15 minutes until it is dark green and crispy. Cool and serve.

KALE SOUP PUREE

🕐 25 MINUTES   3 🍽   VEGAN 🍴

There will be something deeply satisfying—and almost unreal—about your first batch of home-made, pureed green soup. Why should we be so surprised by its shamrock hue? I mean, it's made with fresh kale, right? When kale is pureed, however, and combined with creamy potatoes and zucchini (skin on!), the soup looks even more lively! Sip it slowly, savor it, and know that it will give you a satisfying boost of energy throughout the day.

INGREDIENTS

2 tablespoons extra virgin olive oil

1 shallot, diced

2 garlic cloves

3 medium Yukon gold potatoes, diced

Pinch of sea salt, to taste

Pinch of pepper, to taste

1 zucchini, diced

1 green chile, chopped with seeds removed

6 cups vegetable (or chicken) broth, divided

6 cups baby kale, lightly packed

DIRECTIONS

1. Heat the **olive oil** in a deep pot over medium-high heat. Add the **shallot** and sauté for 2 minutes or until it is translucent. Add the **garlic** and sauté it for another minute or until it becomes fragrant.

2. Add the **potatoes**, sprinkle them with **salt** and **pepper**, and sauté them for about 5–7 minutes or until they are golden brown.

3. Add the **zucchini** and **green chile** and sauté them for another 2 minutes. Add 4 cups of the **broth** and all the **kale**, and simmer for 5–8 minutes until the kale softens and becomes a darker green.

4. Use an immersion blender to blend the soup, or let the soup cool and then transfer it to a blender. Puree the soup for 2 minutes until it is smooth and creamy. Transfer the pureed soup from the blender to the pot on the stove. Stir in the remaining 2 cups of broth. Heat the soup for another 2 minutes, ladle it into bowls, and top it with crispy **Lemon Kale Chips** (page 141).

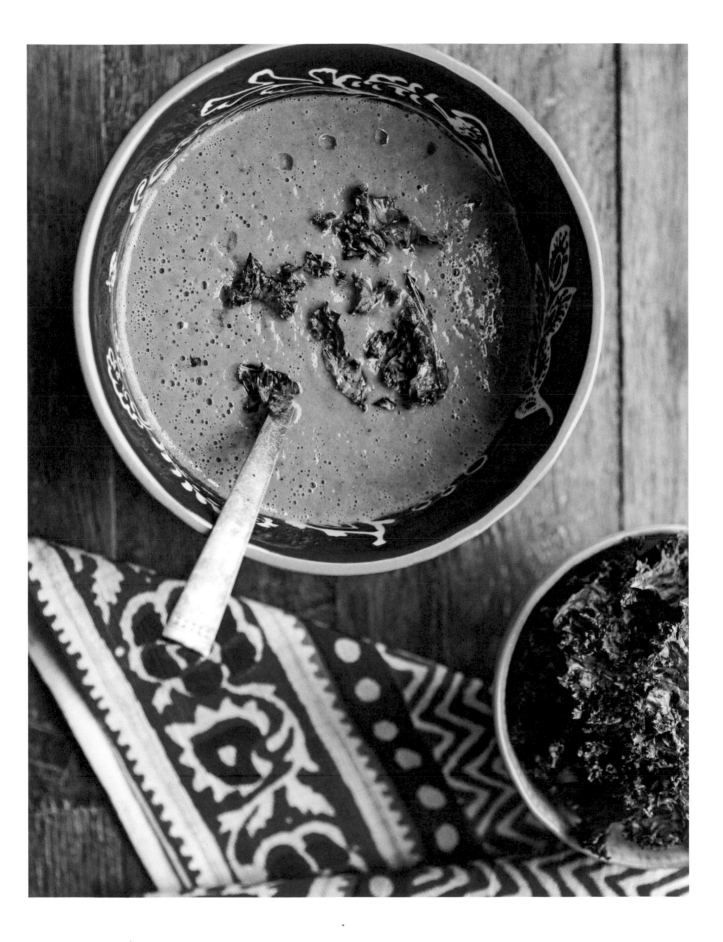

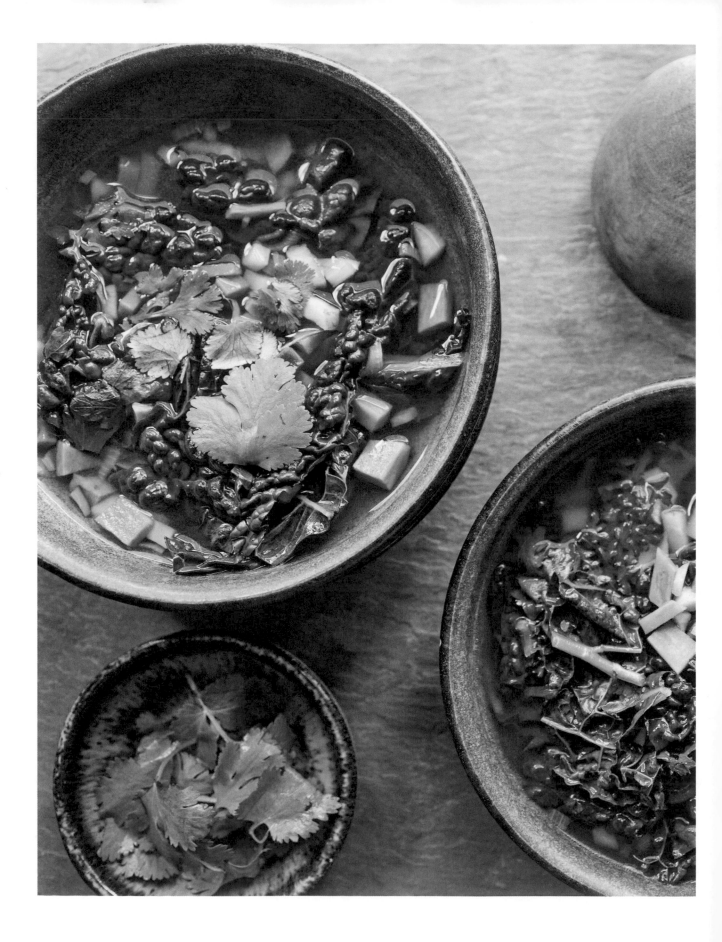

HEARTY KALE SOUP

🕐 20 MINUTES   3 🍽   VEGAN ✗

Although this soup can be eaten at any time of the year, it's one of those nourishing bowls that I love to curl up with on cool autumn days. You can use either curly green or Lacinato (dinosaur) kale in this recipe. What I particularly love about this cruciferous vegetable is that it's not wimpy; it really holds on to a lot of its character, even when it's cooked!

INGREDIENTS

2 tablespoons extra virgin olive oil

1 shallot, diced

2 garlic cloves, diced

1 sweet potato, diced

Pinch of sea salt, to taste

Pinch of pepper, to taste

4 carrots, diced

4 cups vegetable broth, store-bought, or use the recipe for Homemade Vegetable Broth on page 66

1 zucchini, cut and quartered

1 bunch kale, destemmed and chopped

¼ teaspoon crushed red pepper flakes

2 tablespoons cilantro

DIRECTIONS

1. Heat the **olive oil** in a deep pot over medium-high heat. Add the **shallots** and sauté for 2 minutes or until they're translucent. Add the **garlic** and sauté it for another minute or until it becomes fragrant.

2. Add the **sweet potato** and a little **sea salt** and **pepper**, and sauté them for 3–4 minutes. Add the **carrots** and sauté them for another minute.

3. Add the vegetable **broth** to the pot. Raise the heat to high, and bring the soup to a boil. Reduce the heat to a simmer. Add the **zucchini** and let broth simmer for 5 minutes, and then add the **kale** and **red pepper flakes**. Let the soup simmer for another 5 minutes. Season it with salt and pepper to taste. Top with **cilantro** and serve.

KALE SLAW

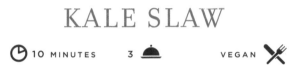

10 MINUTES   3   VEGAN

Coming from both a Polish and German household, cabbage slaw was a popular side dish at lunches and dinners at my grandmother's house. What I love about adding kale to this recipe for slaw is that it transforms it into a main dish from a simple side. Both the cabbage and the kale, which are in the same family of cruciferous vegetables, are nutrient-dense and contain protective compounds, known as glucosinolates, which have been proven to lower cancer risks.

INGREDIENTS

1 bunch kale, destemmed and chopped

2 carrots, peeled and julienned

1 small red cabbage, chopped and thinly sliced

1 shallot, thinly sliced

Pinch of sea salt, to taste

Pinch of pepper, to taste

Juice of 1 lemon

1 tablespoon extra virgin olive oil

2 teaspoons apple cider vinegar (optional)

⅓ cup walnuts (optional)

DIRECTIONS

1. Add the **kale**, **carrots**, **red cabbage**, and **shallot** to a bowl. Toss with some **salt** and **pepper**, the **lemon juice**, and the **olive oil**.

2. If you want to bring in a little more tang to the salad, add the **apple cider vinegar** to the mix. Toss in the **walnuts** if you want an extra nutritious crunch.

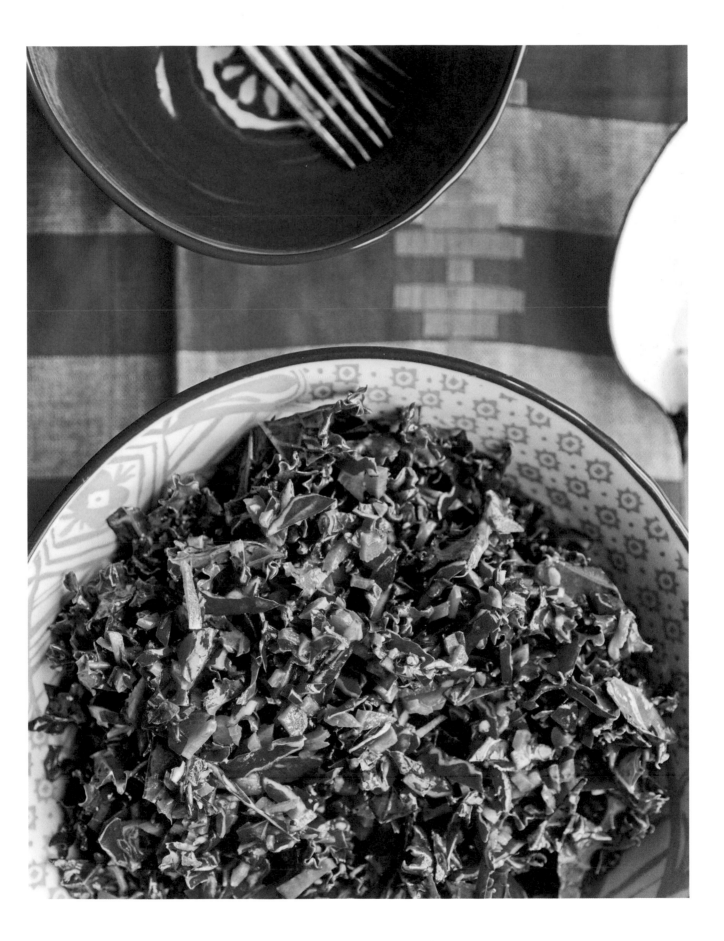

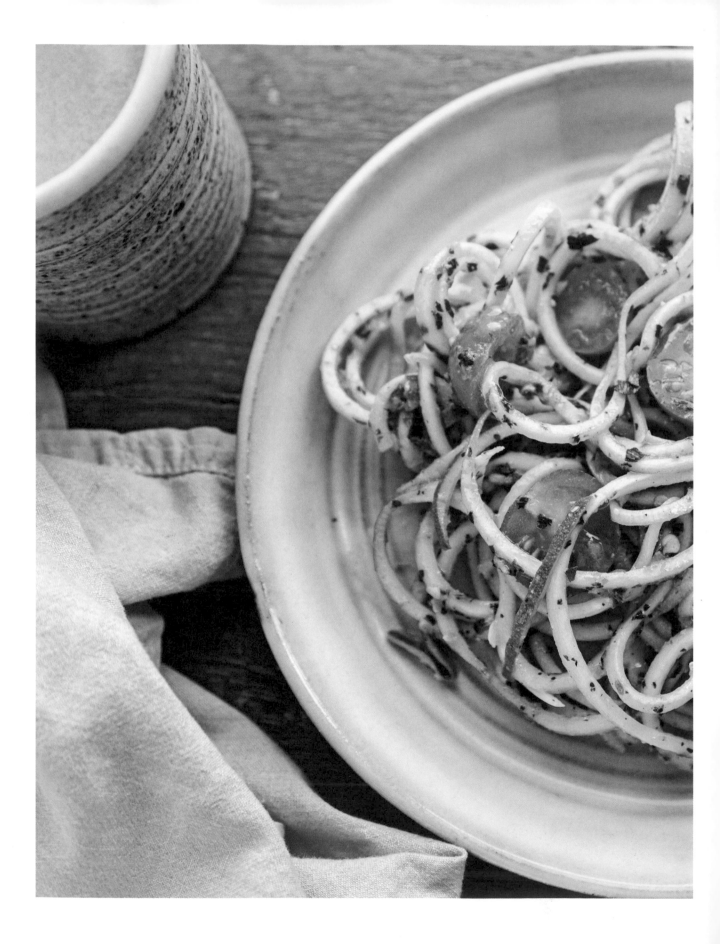

ZUCCHINI NOODLES WITH KALE PESTO AND TOMATOES

🕐 10 MINUTES   3 🍽   VEGAN 🍴

Spiralize some zucchini, make a fresh batch of pesto, roll up your sleeves, and have fun with this simple dish. I've found that zucchini, especially prepped as curly "noodles," holds sauce particularly well, and the slight bitter notes of the kale combined with the sweetness of the tomatoes pull the whole dish together.

INGREDIENTS

2 zucchini

8 cherry tomatoes, sliced

½ bunch kale, destemmed and chopped

¼ cup fresh basil

½ cup walnuts, chopped

2 cloves garlic

½ cup nutritional yeast

¼ cup extra virgin olive oil

Juice of 1 lemon

Pinch of sea salt, to taste

Pinch of pepper, to taste

DIRECTIONS

1. Spiralize the **zucchini** into "noodles" and set them aside in a large bowl along with the **cherry tomatoes**.

2. To make the pesto, bring a medium pot of salted water to a boil. Fill another bowl with **ice** and **water**. Blanch the **kale** for 25 seconds, remove it, and place it in the ice water. Dry the kale in a colander or salad spinner. Combine the kale, **basil**, **walnuts**, **garlic**, **nutritional yeast**, **olive oil**, and **lemon juice** in a blender and blend for 2 minutes or until smooth. Taste and season with **salt** and **pepper**.

3. Mix the kale pesto into the zucchini noodles. Plate and enjoy.

ZUCCHINI, ASPARAGUS, AND PEA SALAD WITH MICROGREENS

🕐 10 MINUTES   2 🍽   VEGAN 🍴

I've made this salad countless times for friends and family. The goodness of each ingredient stands out on its own. The crunchy, mild taste of the zucchini; the grassy, robust taste of an asparagus spear; the sweetness of the peas; and the bite of a savory microgreen mix make this salad a perfect summer meal (though you can easily find these ingredients year-round). Some people like to cut off and compost the tougher, woody stems of the asparagus, but if you want to reduce kitchen waste, you can slice up the stems very finely and add them to the salad.

INGREDIENTS

½ green zucchini

½ yellow zucchini

½ bunch asparagus

½ cup English peas

2 dozen snow peas

1 tablespoon extra virgin olive oil

¼ teaspoon sea salt

⅛ teaspoon pepper

6 ounces microgreen mix

INSTRUCTIONS

1. Slice the **zucchinis** in half. Spiralize the zucchini through a spiralizer to make zucchini noodles, or matchstick them, if you do not have a spiralizer.

2. Blanch the **asparagus, English peas,** and **snow peas** in another saucepan with ½ cup of **water** for about 1 minute or until tender. Drain and set aside.

3. Transfer the zucchini, asparagus, and peas to a bowl and toss the veggies with the **olive oil, salt,** and **pepper**. Top the mixture with the **microgreens** and serve.

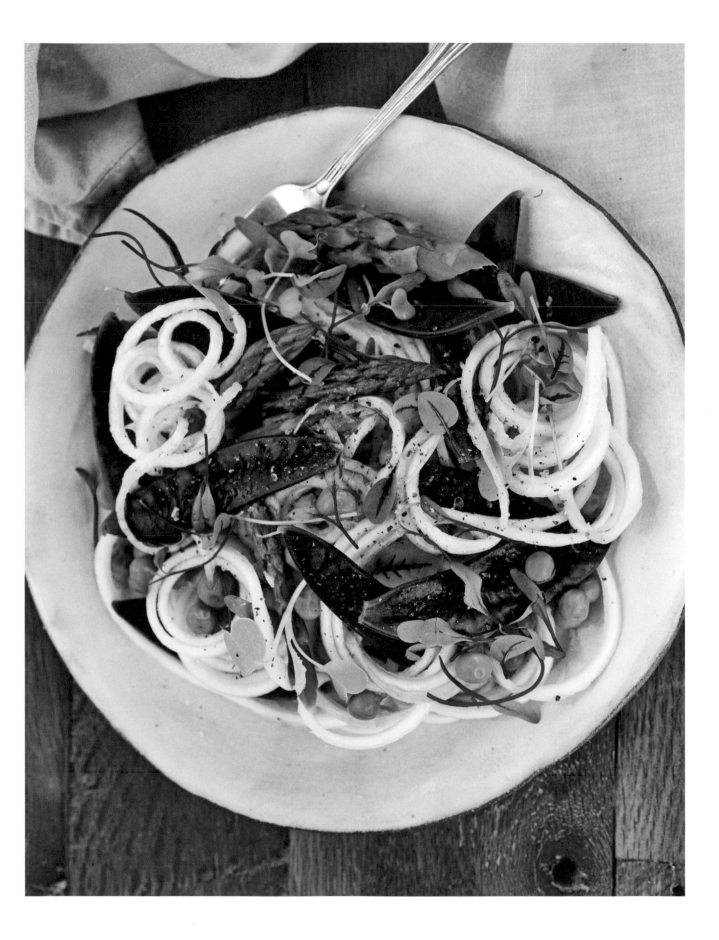

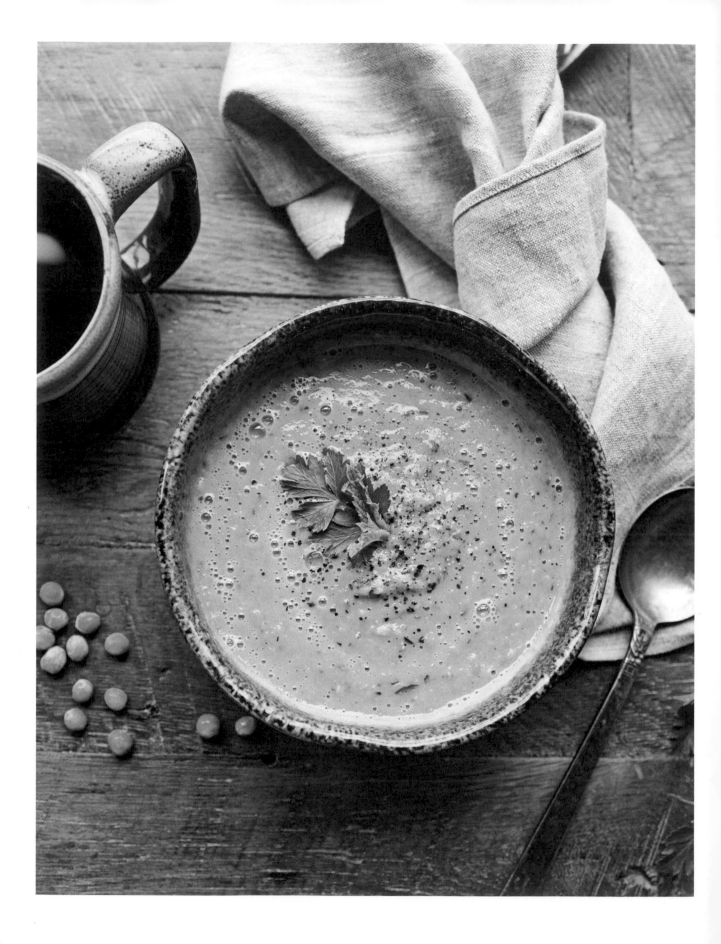

MINTY PEA SOUP

🕐 20 MINUTES   2 🍽   VEGAN ✖

Mint and peas may seem like an unlikely pair, but the combination of the herb's fresh, cleansing taste and the summery sweetness of peas brings out an unusually pleasant flavor that is as bright as the soup itself! Peas are particularly rich in vitamin K, B vitamins, manganese, folate, and an array of antioxidants, which can help reduce inflammation and protect against cancer.

INGREDIENTS

1 tablespoon extra virgin olive oil

½ yellow onion, thinly sliced

1–2 garlic cloves, thinly sliced

1 cup vegetable broth, store-bought, or use the recipe for Homemade Vegetable Broth on page 66

2½ cups English peas

Handful mint leaves, chopped

Handful parsley, chopped

¼ teaspoon sea salt

⅛ teaspoon pepper

DIRECTIONS

1. Heat the **olive oil** in a medium saucepan. Add the **onion** and the **garlic**. Sauté for about two minutes or until fragrant.

2. Add the vegetable **broth** and the **peas**. Bring the mixture to a light boil, and then simmer for 5 minutes.

3. Remove the saucepan from the heat. Add both the **mint** and the **parsley** and stir. Blend the soup in a blender or with an immersion blender. Add ½ cup of **water** or more, depending on how thick you like your soup. Add **salt** and **pepper** as needed.

BAKED LEMON-THYME SOLE WITH ZUCCHINI, ASPARAGUS, AND PEA SALAD

🕐 **20** MINUTES   **2** 🍽   PESCATARIAN 🐟

Sole is a most agreeable fish, because its luscious white flesh is so mild; even my non–fish loving friends will wolf down lemony sole. It's also a particularly thin fish, so it cooks in no time at all, and it takes on the flavor of whatever you dress it up with—in this case, a little lemon and lemon zest, which go a long way.

INGREDIENTS

1 lemon

2 sole fillets

½ teaspoon sea salt

¼ teaspoon ground black pepper

1 tablespoon extra virgin olive oil

1 shallot, minced

1 cup English peas

½ bunch asparagus

½ green zucchini

Handful of thyme

DIRECTIONS

1. Zest the **lemon** and set aside the zest.

2. Place the **sole fillets** in a glass baking dish. Rub the fillets with **salt**, **pepper**, and a squeeze of **lemon juice**. Cut the lemon in round slices and place them on top of the fillets. If you have the time, let the fish marinate in the refrigerator for 20–30 minutes. Otherwise, place it in the oven at 350°F for 15 minutes or until the flesh flakes easily with a fork.

3. Heat the **olive oil** over medium heat in a nonstick skillet. Add the **shallot** and sauté it for 2 minutes or until translucent. Add the **peas**, **asparagus**, and **zucchini** to the skillet and sauté for about 3 minutes or until they are tender. Remove the veggies from the heat and plate them.

4. Remove the fillets from the oven. Plate them, and season with **fresh thyme**, salt, pepper, and 1 tablespoon of the lemon zest (reserve the remaining zest for another use).

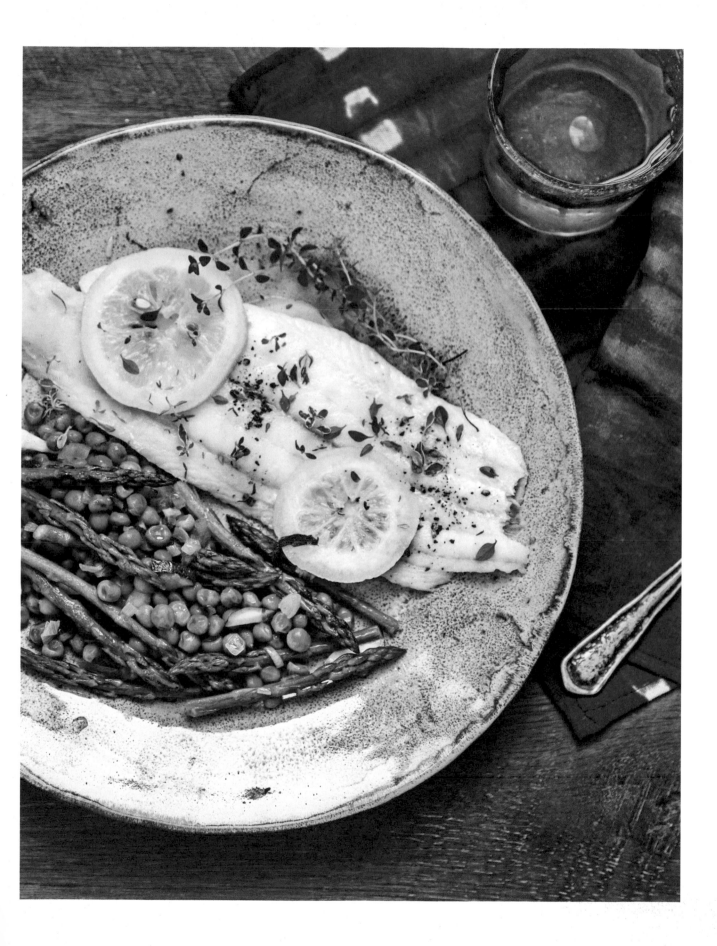

MEAL MAP 6

HAVE **29** PANTRY STAPLES READY AND SHOP FOR THESE **9** MAIN INGREDIENTS
TO MAKE **7** RECIPES AND **25** SERVINGS OF FOOD.

RECIPES

INGREDIENTS

2 heads cauliflower

1 small head broccoli

2 butternut squash

2 bunches carrots

1 banana

8 cups kale

4 pastured eggs

1 pound shrimp

2⅓ 13.5-ounce cans coconut
milk

PANTRY STAPLES

Red Onion × 1

Shallots × 2

Ginger × 1

Garlic × 1

Yellow onion × 1

Limes × 2

Lemons × 3

Sea salt

Pepper

Extra virgin olive oil

Le Puy lentils

Vegetable or chicken broth

White wine vinegar

Sherry vinegar

Thyme

Cilantro

Nutmeg

Cinnamon

Vanilla extract

Carob powder

Curry powder

Turmeric

Cumin

Cayenne pepper

Bay leaves

Coconut oil

Coconut flour

Pomegranate seeds

Peppercorns

OPTIONAL

Microgreens

Kefir

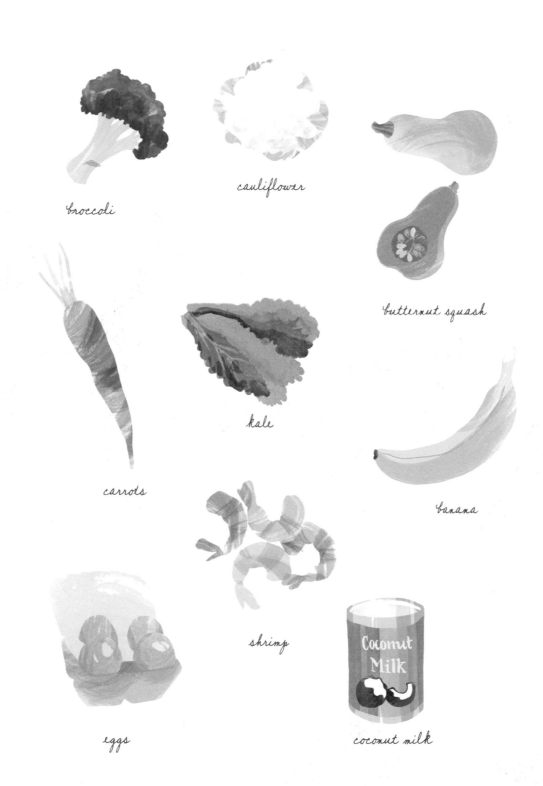

broccoli

cauliflower

butternut squash

carrots

kale

banana

shrimp

eggs

Coconut Milk

coconut milk

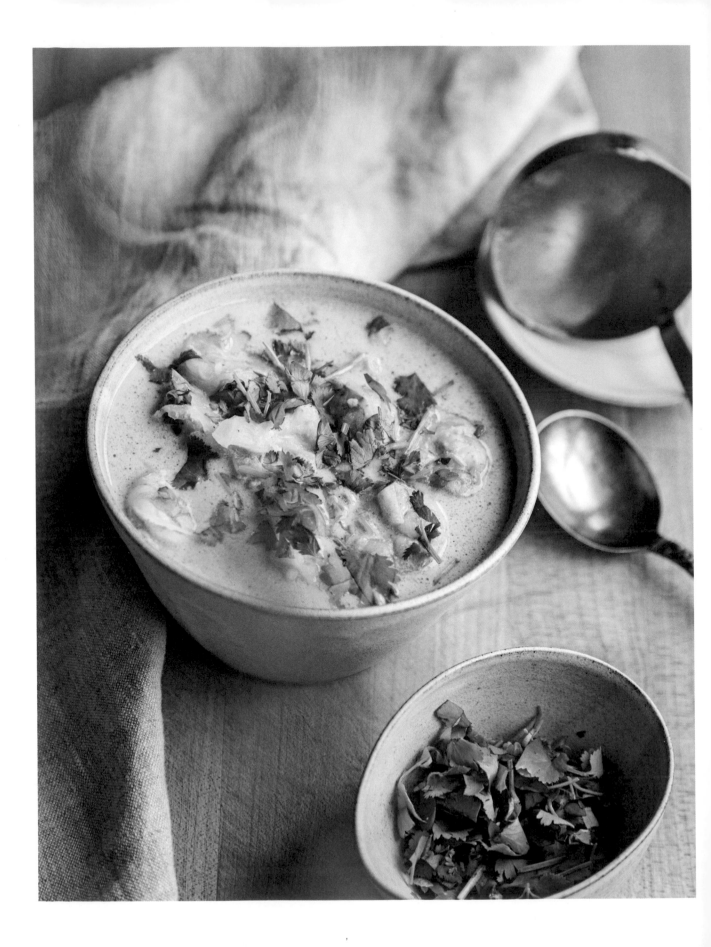

COCONUT-CURRY SHRIMP SOUP

🕐 10 MINUTES　　2 🍽　　PESCATARIAN 🐟

When I first decided to do a sugar cleanse, I let all my friends know why I was doing it and invited everyone to have dinner at my house over the course of the next few weeks. Who can say no to that! That's when I first concocted this recipe for an all-ladies' get-together. I wanted something that I could make in a big batch that was light and mouth-wateringly flavorful. Using fresh spices and herbs is particularly appealing when you're removing sugar from your diet because it gives real flavor to food and reorients your taste buds to what real food tastes like. Everyone said, "Wow, what's *this* recipe!?!" Goal achieved!

INGREDIENTS

1 shallot, diced

1 tablespoon extra virgin olive oil

2 tablespoons ginger

1 tablespoon curry powder

1 teaspoon turmeric

½ teaspoon cumin

2 13.5-ounce cans coconut milk

2 cups vegetable broth, store-bought, or use the recipe for Homemade Vegetable Broth on page 66

1 cauliflower, finely chopped

1 pound shrimp, cleaned and deveined

Pinch of sea salt, to taste

2 tablespoons cilantro (optional)

1 ounce microgreens (optional)

DIRECTIONS

1. Sauté the **shallot** in a pan with the **olive oil** until it's translucent, about 2 minutes. Add the **ginger** to the mix and continue until the shallot is caramelized.

2. Once the shallot is caramelized, add the **curry powder**, **turmeric**, and **cumin**.

3. Add the **coconut milk** and vegetable **broth** to the mixture and bring to a simmer. Then add the **cauliflower** and **shrimp** and cook for another 2 minutes, or until the shrimp is pink. Add **salt** to taste.

4. Take the pan off the stove and add some **cilantro** and **microgreens** as a garnish.

ROASTED CURRIED CAULIFLOWER WITH LENTILS AND QUICK-PICKLED ONIONS

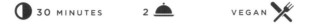

◑ 30 MINUTES   2 🍽   VEGAN 🍴

Unlike other legumes, which can take quite a bit of preparation time, lentils can be made very easily. They are particularly high in both insoluble and soluble fiber, too, which means that they prevent blood sugar levels from spiking after a meal. A general rule of thumb is that brown, black, and green lentils (the ones suggested in this recipe) are better at holding their shape ("green, brown, black bounce back"), whereas the yellow, orange, and red typically turn mushy; the latter are much better for thickening soups and making dal, a popular Indian dish.

INGREDIENTS

1 cup Le Puy lentils

1 bay leaf

1 head cauliflower, destemmed, florets chopped

2 tablespoons extra virgin olive oil

1 tablespoon curry powder

Pinch of salt

Pinch of pepper

Juice of 1 lemon

Pinch of cayenne pepper, to taste

⅓ cup quick pickled onions (see page 159)

¼ cup fresh cilantro leaves

1 tablespoon pomegranate seeds

DIRECTIONS

1. Rinse the **lentils** with cold water in a colander or fine mesh sieve to remove any debris. Add the lentils to at least 3 cups of fresh **water** in a medium saucepan. Toss a **bay leaf** into the saucepan and add a pinch of **salt**. Bring the water to a boil and then reduce the heat and simmer for 20–25 minutes.

2. Preheat the oven to 450°F. In a large bowl, toss the **cauliflower** florets together with the **olive oil**, **curry powder**, salt, and **pepper**. For an added kick, drizzle some **lemon juice** over the mixture and sprinkle it with a pinch of **cayenne pepper**.

3. Spread the cauliflower mixture in a single layer over a large baking pan. Bake it for about 25 minutes or until the cauliflower is tender and begins to turn a golden brown.

4. Add some **quick-pickled onions** to the cauliflower, and garnish it with **fresh cilantro** and some **pomegranate seeds**.

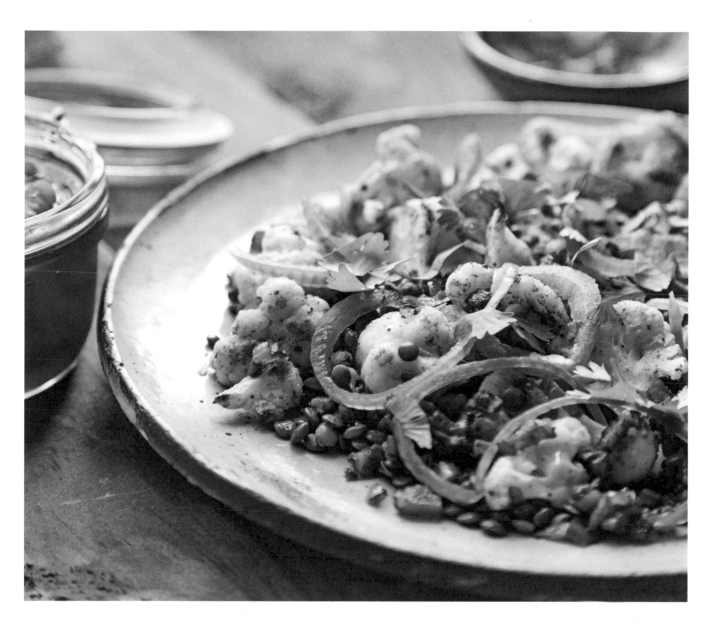

FOR QUICK-PICKLED ONIONS

INGREDIENTS

1 small red onion

1 small clove garlic, peeled

3 red, white, or black peppercorns

2 small sprigs of thyme

½ teaspoon salt

⅔ cup white wine vinegar

DIRECTIONS

1. Peel and then slice the **onion** into thin moon shapes. Add the onion, **garlic**, **peppercorns**, and **thyme** to a mason jar.

2. Whisk the **salt** and **vinegar** together in a small bowl. Pour the mixture into the jar, making sure to cover the onions with the liquid. Let the onion mixture sit in the jar for about 30 minutes, then chill it in the refrigerator. The onions will keep for 2 weeks.

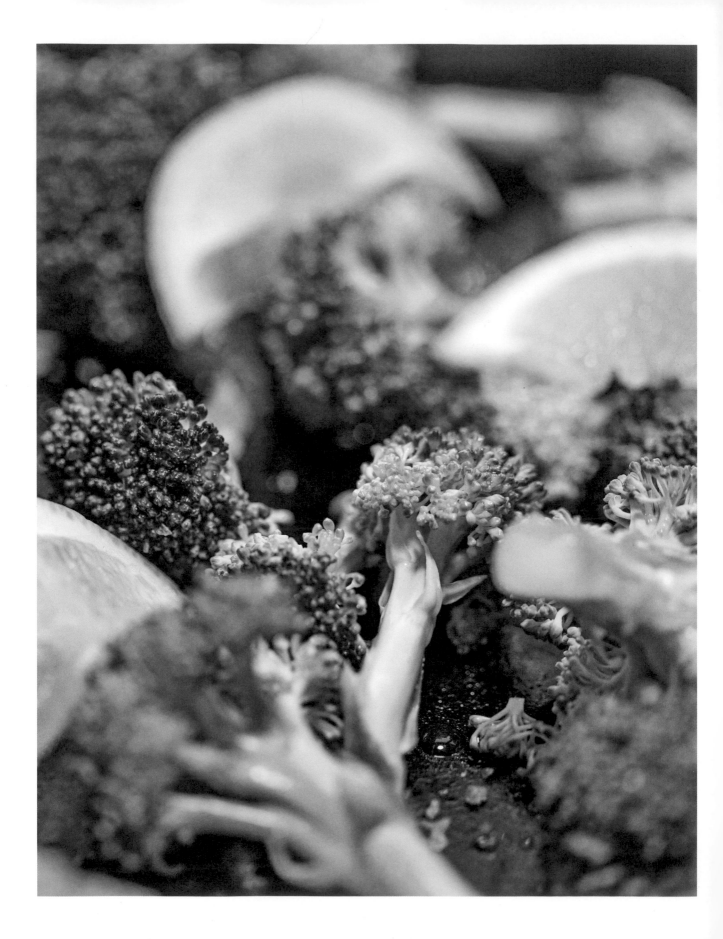

CHARRED BROCCOLI WITH LEMON PEEL

🕐 25 MINUTES   4 🍽   VEGAN ✗

Broccoli, like its early cabbage ancestors, is a powerhouse of nutrients. Both the compact florets and fibrous stems are packed full of vitamins, minerals, and cancer-fighting compounds, including lutein and glucosinolates like indole-3-carbinole and sulforaphane. Raw broccoli can be unappetizing for some people, but dressed in a little olive oil, lemon juice, and a pinch of salt, it can be radically transformed into an all-around sensational dish.

INGREDIENTS

1 head broccoli, cut into florets

2 tablespoons extra virgin olive oil

Juice of 1 lemon, divided

⅛ teaspoon of sea salt

½ lemon, thinly sliced

DIRECTIONS

1. Preheat the oven to 425°F.

2. Toss the **broccoli** in a large bowl with the **olive oil**, half the **lemon juice**, and a sprinkle of **salt**. Spread the florets on a baking sheet and add the **lemon peel** to the broccoli. Roast the florets for 15 minutes.

3. Remove the baking sheet from the oven and sprinkle the remaining lemon juice over the broccoli. Bake it for another 5 minutes and serve.

GINGERED CARROT AND BUTTERNUT SQUASH SOUP

⬤◐ 90 MINUTES   4 🍽   VEGAN ✕

The bright orange color of carrots and squash is due to beta-carotene, which, as my mother always reminded me as a child, is good for your eyesight. Beta-carotene, which appropriately derives its name from *carrot*, is the precursor for vitamin A, which is essential for the health of our skin, mucus membranes, immune system, and, yes, our vision. One of my favorite ingredients in any soup my mother made was the carrot, perhaps due to its natural sweetness. I love carrots so much that I always encouraged my mother to add another bunch or bag.

INGREDIENTS

1 butternut squash, peeled, cubed, and seeded

3 tablespoons extra virgin olive oil, divided

2 cups carrots, peeled

1 yellow onion, finely diced

2 tablespoons fresh ginger, peeled and grated (more if you like real zing!)

2 cloves garlic, crushed

6 cups vegetable (or chicken) broth

¼ teaspoon ground nutmeg

¼ teaspoon ground cinnamon

¼ teaspoon sea salt

¼ teaspoon ground white or red pepper

DIRECTIONS

1. Preheat the oven to 375°F.

2. Toss the **butternut squash** and **carrots** in a large bowl in 2½ tablespoons of the **olive oil**. Put them in a parchment-lined baking dish, and bake for about 45 minutes or until they are nicely browned and tender. Remove the baking dish from the oven.

3. In a large pot, heat the remaining ½ tablespoon of olive oil over medium heat. Add the **onion** and cook it for about 5 minutes until it is translucent. Add the **ginger** and **garlic** to the pot and cook them for 1 minute. Add the squash, **carrots**, **broth**, **nutmeg**, **cinnamon**, **salt**, and **pepper** to the pot. Bring the mixture to boil by increasing the heat to medium-high. Reduce the heat to low and simmer the mix, uncovered, for about 30 minutes.

4. Remove the pot from the heat and let the mixture cool slightly. Blend it with an immersion blender or transfer the soup in batches to a blender and puree it until the soup is creamy. Add more salt and pepper to taste.

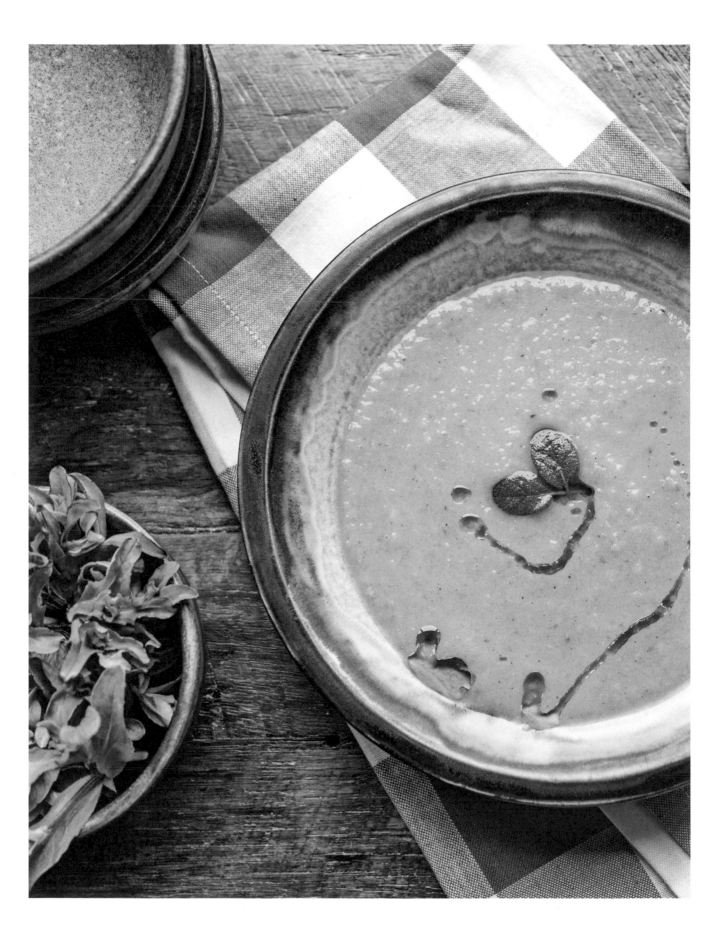

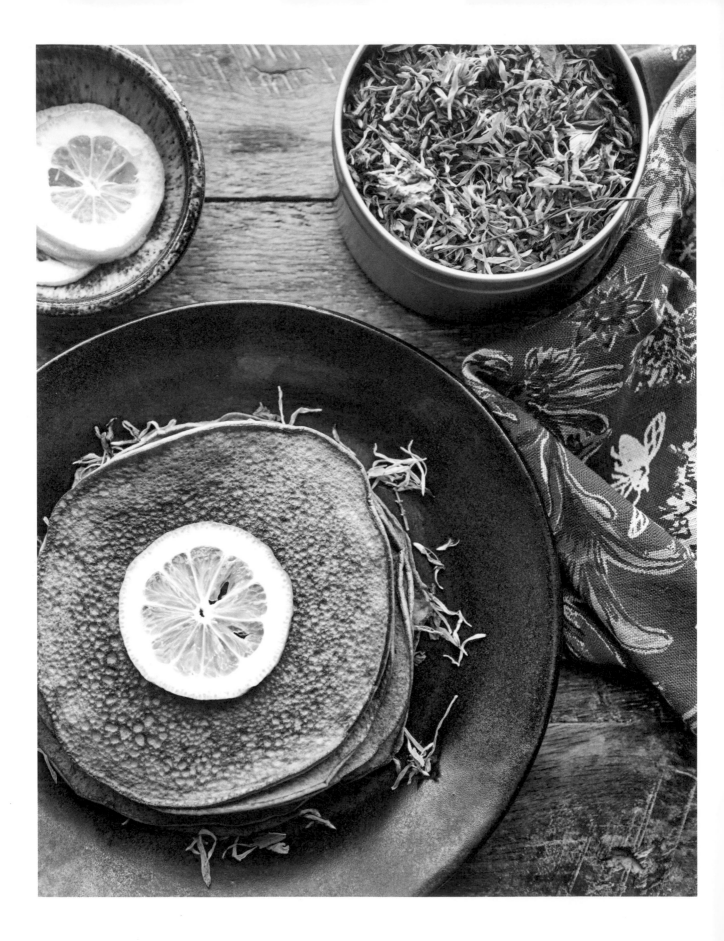

COCONUT PANCAKES

🕐 15 MINUTES   5 🍽   VEGETARIAN 🌿

Part of going through a sugar cleanse involves reacclimating your taste buds to foods that are naturally sweet. These coconut pancakes fit the bill and are seriously satisfying.

INGREDIENTS

1 small banana

4 eggs

¼ cup coconut flour, plus additional as needed

⅓ cup canned coconut milk (try to use just the coconut cream)

1 teaspoon vanilla

1 teaspoon carob powder

1 teaspoon cinnamon

1 tablespoon coconut oil

Squeeze of lemon juice

1 cup kefir (optional)

DIRECTIONS

1. Add the **banana** and **eggs** to a blender and blend on low. Add the **coconut flour**, then the **coconut milk**, **vanilla**, **carob powder**, and **cinnamon**. Blend until well mixed. If the mixture is too liquid, add 1 more tablespoon of the coconut flour.

2. Heat the **coconut oil** in a skillet over low to medium heat. Slowly pour 3–4 tablespoons of the mixture into the hot skillet per pancake. Heat the pancakes until bubbles start to form, about 2 minutes, then flip them and let them brown lightly on the other side. Squeeze a little **lemon juice** on top of each pancake. Serve the pancakes with **kefir** for added flavor.

GINGER-LIME KALE SALAD WITH LENTILS AND BUTTERNUT SQUASH

🕐 35 MINUTES   4 🍽   VEGAN 🍴

Warm salads may not sound appetizing at first, but kale is quite a hearty leaf, and working out some of its toughness can be done several ways: lightly sautéing it just as it starts to soften, for example. In this dish, the kale is deliciously paired with nutrient-dense lentils and sweet, buttery winter squash.

INGREDIENTS

½ cup Le Puy lentils

1 bay leaf

¼ teaspoon sea salt, divided

½ medium butternut squash, peeled, seeded, and cubed

2 tablespoons extra virgin olive oil, divided

1 shallot, diced

2 cloves garlic, minced

1 tablespoon fresh ginger, peeled and grated (more if you like real zing!)

8 cups kale leaves, destemmed and thinly sliced

1 tablespoon fresh lime juice

DIRECTIONS

1. Rinse the **lentils** with cold water in a colander or fine mesh sieve to remove any debris. Add the lentils to at least 2 cups of fresh **water** in a medium saucepan. Toss in a **bay leaf** and some **salt**. Bring the mixture to a boil and then reduce the heat and simmer for 20–25 minutes. Drain the mixture, cover it, and set it aside.

2. Preheat the oven to 400°F. In a large bowl, toss the **squash** with 1 tablespoon of the **olive oil**. Spread the squash onto a parchment-lined baking sheet and roast it for about 25 minutes, or until the squash is firm but tender and can be pierced with a fork. Remove the squash from the oven and let it cool.

3. While the lentils are simmering and the squash is roasting, heat a wide and deep skillet over medium-low heat. Add the remaining 1 tablespoon of olive oil to coat the skillet. Add the **shallot** and cook it for 2 minutes or until it's translucent. Add the **garlic** and **ginger**, stirring for another minute.

4. Add the **kale** and cook, stirring, for about 2 minutes, until the kale begins to wilt. Remove the pan from the heat. Plate the kale and top it with the squash, lentils, **lime juice**, and salt. Serve and enjoy.

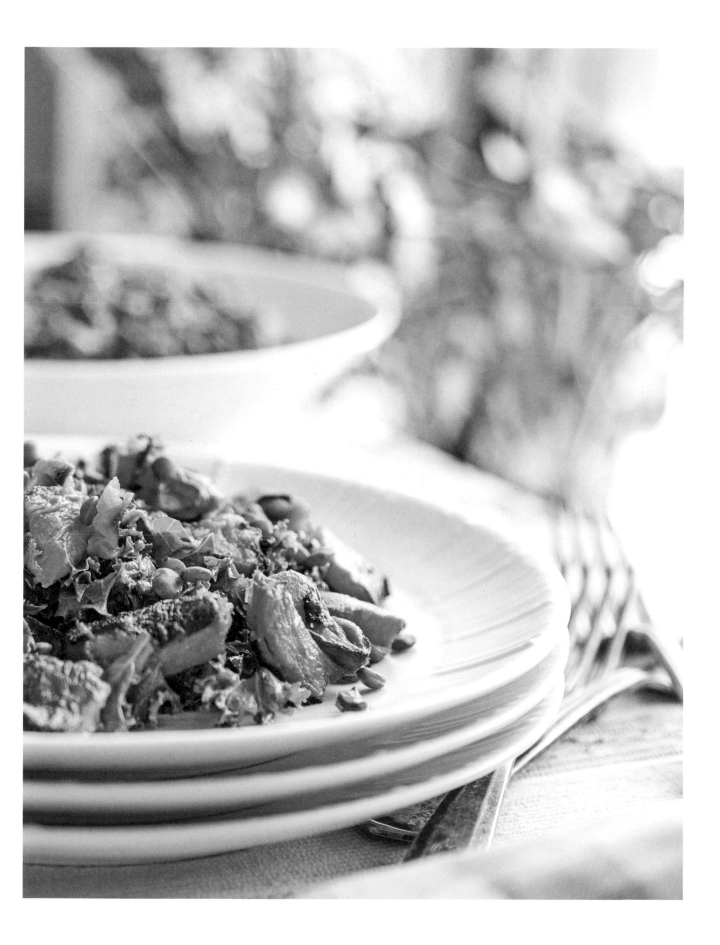

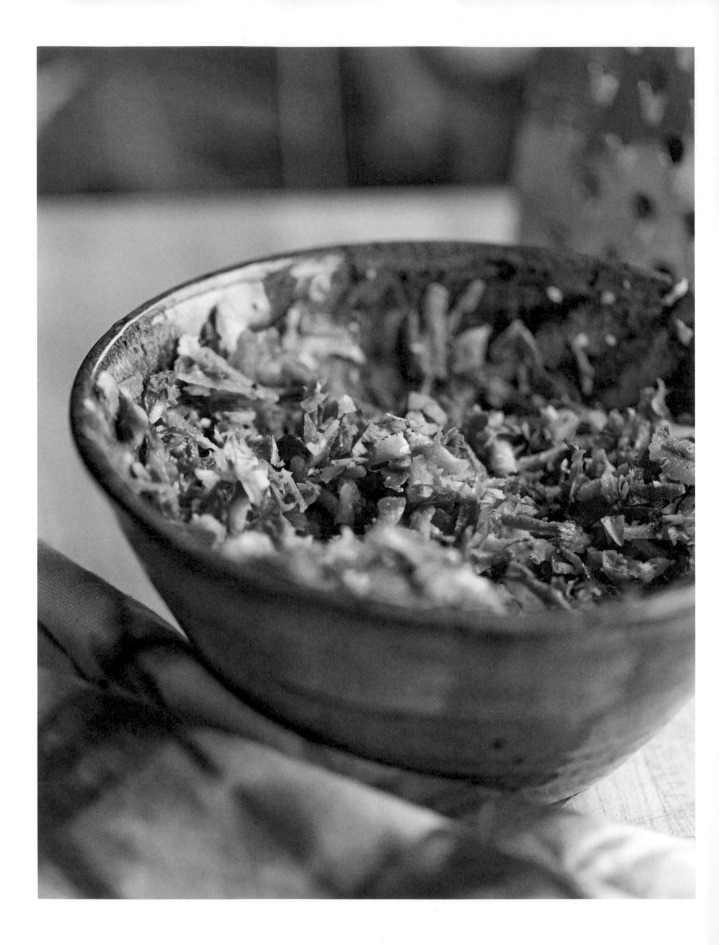

GINGERED CARROT SALAD

20 MINUTES   4   VEGAN

Carrots, raw and undressed, are one of those vegetables that are fun and easy to eat. Shredding them can offer a new experience, though, and the vinegar and ginger in this recipe tease out the juiciest of flavors, giving the carrot a zesty new twist.

INGREDIENTS

2 cups shredded carrots

1 garlic clove, peeled and grated

1 tablespoon sherry vinegar

1 tablespoon fresh ginger

½ cup cilantro, coarsely chopped, divided

1 tablespoon extra virgin olive oil, divided

¼ teaspoon sea salt

⅛ teaspoon freshly ground pepper

1 teaspoon lime juice

DIRECTIONS

1. In a medium bowl, toss the **carrots** with the **garlic**, **vinegar**, **ginger**, ¼ cup of the **cilantro**, and 1 tablespoon of the **olive oil**. Season the carrots with **salt** and **pepper**. Let the carrots stand for 15 minutes, then drain them well.

2. Add the **lime juice** and the remaining ¼ cup of **cilantro** to the carrots and toss well. Transfer the salad to a bowl and serve.

MEAL MAP 7

Have 17 pantry staples ready and shop for these 14 main ingredients to make 8 recipes and 26 servings.

RECIPES

INGREDIENTS

5-6 heads small green cabbage

2 bunches kale

4 small potatoes

2 bunches carrots

4 parsnips

1 16-ounce jar sauerkraut

1 13.5-ounce can coconut milk

9 pastured eggs

4 cups tomato sauce or strained tomato soup

1 6-ounce can tomato paste

1 32-ounce can San Marzano tomatoes

2 pounds cooked ham

1 pound ground pork

2 pounds Polska kielbasa

PANTRY STAPLES

Shallots × 7

Yellow onions × 3

Garlic × 2

Lemon × 1

Pearl barley

Sea salt

Pepper

Extra virgin olive oil

Cumin

Rice wine vinegar

Paprika

Rosemary

Parsley

Dill

Bay leaves

Coconut oil

Vegetable stock

OPTIONAL

Crushed red pepper

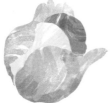

green cabbage

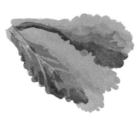

kale

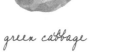

potatoes

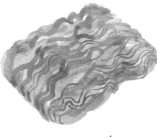

carrots

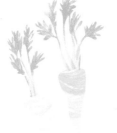

parsnips

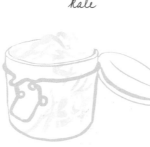

sauerkraut

coconut milk

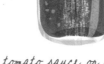

eggs

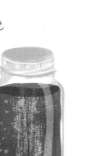

tomato sauce or strained
tomato soup

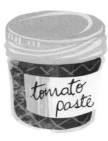

tomato paste

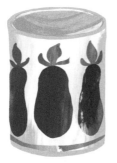

San Marzano tomatoes

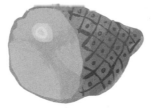

cooked ham

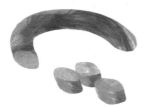

ground pork

Polska kielbasa

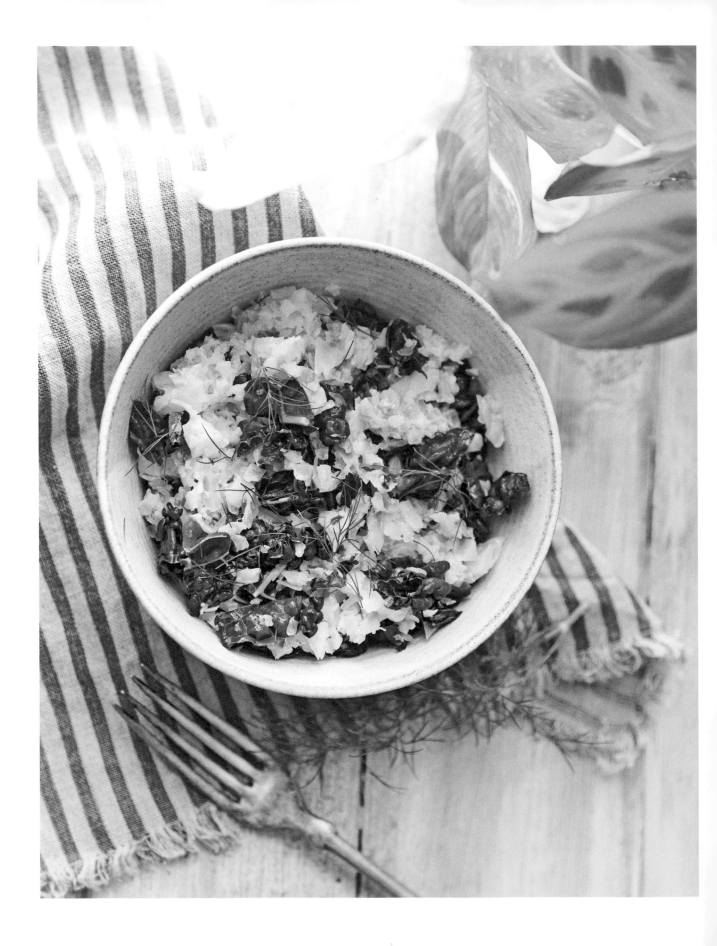

CABBAGE AND KALE MASH

🕐 15 MINUTES   2 🍽   VEGAN 🍴

Cabbage can look intimidating. Most varieties can grow quite large (think bowling balls); they are compact, dense, and relatively heavy; and if you don't know what to do with a whole head, you might find yourself wasting quite a bit of good food. Raw cabbage leaves are quite thick and have a rubbery texture; cooking them down softens them and releases a lot of their water content (a cabbage is 96 percent water). The cabbage and kale mash in this dish is akin to mashed potatoes and can easily be served as a side or, because it's so filling, a whole meal.

INGREDIENTS

4 cups washed and chopped green cabbage

1 tablespoon coconut oil

1 shallot

2 tablespoons coconut cream (separated from the milk)

½ teaspoon cumin

1 cup kale, destemmed and finely chopped

1 tablespoon parsley, chopped

Pinch fresh dill

Juice of ½ lemon

Pinch of sea salt, to taste

DIRECTIONS

1. Boil the **cabbage** in 1 cup of **salted water** and let it cook for 3–4 minutes. Drain the cabbage.

2. Heat the **coconut oil** in a nonstick skillet and sauté the **shallot** over low heat for 2 minutes or until it is translucent. Add the drained cabbage, **coconut cream**, and **cumin**. Cover and cook the cabbage mixture for about 8 minutes.

3. When the cabbage leaves have become supple, add the **kale**, **parsley**, **dill**, the **lemon juice**, and **salt**. Mix and cook the mixture for a few more minutes.

CABBAGE AND HAM SOUP

🕐 55 MINUTES   5 🍽   NON-VEGETARIAN 🍽

Growing up with a Polish great-grandmother and grandmother, you'd be hard-pressed *not* to find cabbage growing in the garden or on the dinner table. Cabbage and ham soup is a popular meal in my family. We'd eat it for days after special occasions, like Easter, when the roasted ham had been served. "You just toss in any leftover parts—bones, meat, and all into the soup stock," my grandmother said, offering her thoughts on the re-creation of the recipe. "And you can use the ham bone for several times afterwards"—a testament to scrappier times when a person could appreciate the mileage to be had from one item of food.

INGREDIENTS

2 tablespoons extra virgin olive oil

1 medium yellow onion, chopped

4 cloves garlic, minced

1 small cabbage, stem removed and chopped

4 carrots, chopped

16 ounces sauerkraut

1 pound cooked ham, cubed

10 cups vegetable broth, store-bought, or use the recipe for Homemade Vegetable Broth on page 66

2 bay leaves

Pinch of black pepper, to taste

DIRECTIONS

1. Heat the **olive oil** in a deep pot over medium-high heat. Sauté the **onion** for 3 minutes. Sauté the **garlic** for another 2 minutes.

2. Add the **cabbage**, **carrots**, **sauerkraut**, and **ham** to the pot. Cook for 3–5 minutes, stirring frequently.

3. Pour the **broth** into the pot. Add the **bay leaves**. Allow the broth to come to a simmer partially covered for about 40 minutes. Season the soup to taste with some **black pepper**. Remove the bay leaves and serve.

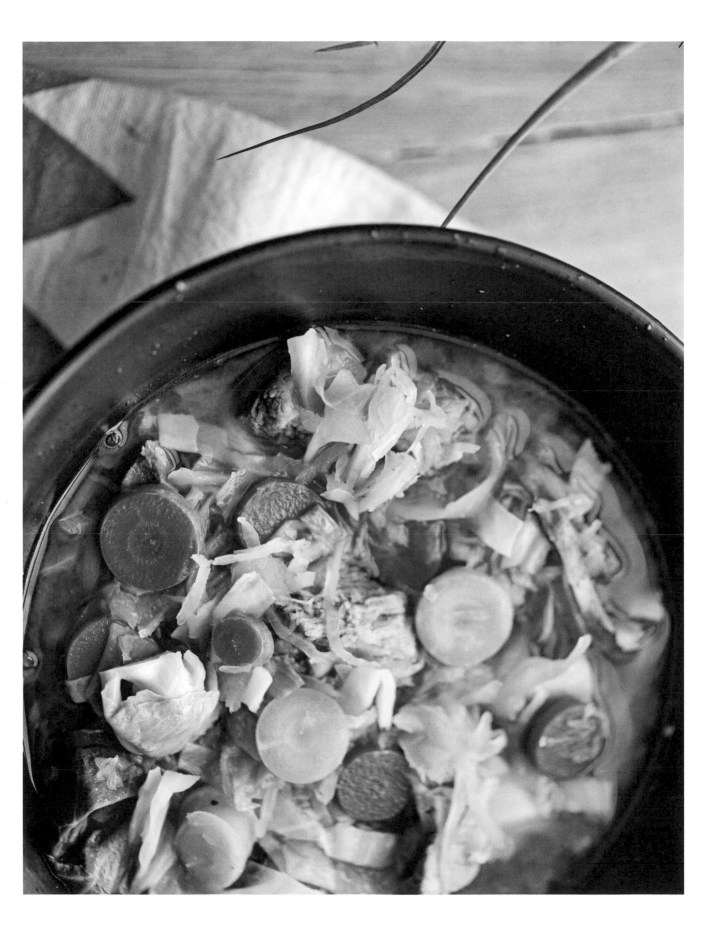

SKILLET CABBAGE WITH KIELBASA

🕐 15 MINUTES   2 🍽   NON-VEGETARIAN 🍴

In Pennsylvania, I grew up near one of the best local kielbasa houses, which meant that we always had access to good Polish sausage. It wasn't something we ate often, except around the holidays, so whenever we had leftovers, we'd either eat the kielbasa cold or sauté it with any leftover veggies, including cabbage. A quick tip on cabbage storage: In the supermarket, cabbage generally comes in perforated plastic bags, which helps the cabbage stay good for a couple of weeks, but once you cut into the cabbage, it typically loses its vitamin C content quite rapidly. So even though it'll stay fresh-looking for a long time, try to use cabbage within a couple of days of cutting it if you want the optimum nutritional benefits.

INGREDIENTS

1½ teaspoons extra virgin olive oil

1 pound fully cooked Polska kielbasa, cut into half moons

1 small head cabbage, coarsely chopped

2 shallots, diced

1 clove garlic, minced

Pinch of pepper

DIRECTIONS

1. Heat the **olive oil** in a large nonstick skillet over medium-high heat. Add the **kielbasa** and cook for 3 minutes, stirring occasionally. Transfer to a plate.

2. In the same pan with some of the fat, add the **cabbage**, **shallot**, **garlic**, and **pepper**. Stir to combine and cook for about 8 minutes, stirring occasionally. Serve.

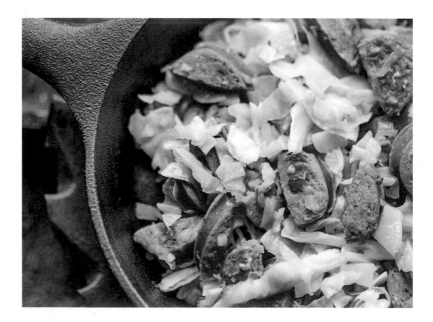

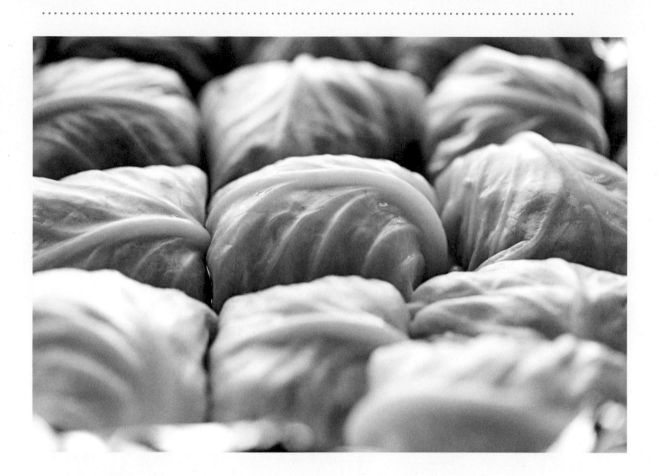

HOW TO SCORE A CABBAGE

When using individual cabbage leaves for holubce, you'll want to make sure they tear off easily after boiling. First make incisions around the core of the cabbage, making sure not to cut entirely through. Once you boil the cabbage and the leaves become soft and pliable, you will be able to remove the leaves more easily.

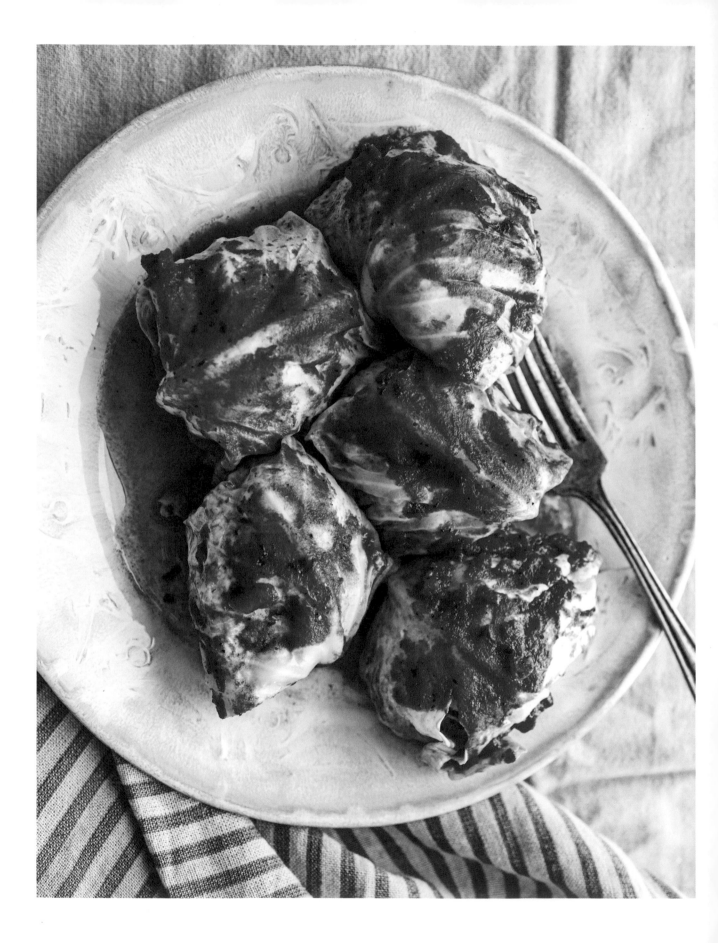

GRANDMA'S HOLUBCE

● ⏱ 105 MINUTES　　🍽 6　　NON-VEGETARIAN 🍴

Of my grandmother's dishes, this one has always been my favorite. When I would come over, she'd ask, "What would you like to eat?" I would enthusiastically say, "Pigs in the blanket," which is what we'd call *holubce*, or what some folks refer to as *golabki*. I thought the name was appropriate, because *holubce* is basically composed of balls of meat, typically pork (though my grandmother later made them with ground turkey), wrapped in a supple "blanket" of cabbage leaves and baked in a tomato sauce. This recipe is true to my family recipe, except I substituted pearl barley for the usual white rice, which gives a similar chewy consistency but adds more nutrients and a nuttier flavor.

INGREDIENTS

1 cup pearled barley

2½ cups vegetable broth, store-bought, or use the recipe for Homemade Vegetable Broth on page 66

1 medium head cabbage

1 pound ground pork

2 cloves garlic, minced

1 small yellow onion, diced

1 egg

Pinch of sea salt

Pinch of pepper

4 cups tomato sauce (homemade is best) or strained tomato soup

1 tablespoon rice wine vinegar

DIRECTIONS

1. Bring the **barley** and **vegetable broth** to a boil. Reduce the heat to a simmer, and cook the barley, covered, until it is tender and most of the liquid has been absorbed, about 45 minutes. (If you are cooking the barley in a pressure cooker, cook it for 18 minutes.) Drain the barley.

2. Score the bottom of the **cabbage** with four 2 inch (5 centimeter) incisions lengthwise, but don't cut all the way through the stem, as we want the leaves to still remain on while boiling. Place the cabbage in a deep pot over high heat and add water to cover. Boil the cabbage for about 15 minutes or until it is pliable. Drain and cool the cabbage. Remove the whole leaves and set them aside.

3. In a separate large bowl, combine the **pork**, barley, **garlic**, **onion**, **egg**, **salt**, and **pepper**, mixing well. Place a small amount of the mixture—about the size of your palm—into the center of a cabbage leaf and fold the leaf over, tucking in the sides of the leaf to keep the meat mixture inside. Place the filled leaves in a baking pan.

4. Preheat the oven to 350°F. Combine the **tomato sauce** and **vinegar** and pour the mixture over the top of the cabbage rolls. Cover the pan with foil and bake for 1 hour.

SMOKY TOMATO SOUP WITH KALE

🕐 40 MINUTES   🍽 2   VEGAN 🍴

Although this recipe calls for canned tomatoes, you can use fresh tomatoes, if you grow your own or buy them from a farmers market in season (June through October in the Northeast). If you use fresh tomatoes, core the stems, boil the tomatoes for 1 minute until skin starts to peel and wrinkle, plunge them in ice water, and then remove the skins before pureeing.

INGREDIENTS

2 tablespoons extra virgin olive oil

1 shallot, diced

2 cloves garlic, minced

2 tablespoons tomato paste

½ tablespoon smoked paprika

½ teaspoon cumin

4 cups (1 32-ounce can) San Marzano tomatoes

2 cups vegetable broth, store-bought, or use the recipe for Homemade Vegetable Broth on page 66

Pinch of sea salt, to taste

Pinch of pepper, to taste

1 bunch kale, destemmed and ribboned

Pinch of crushed red pepper flakes (optional)

DIRECTIONS

1. Heat the **olive oil** in a deep pot over medium heat and sauté the **shallot** for 2 minutes or until it is translucent. Add the **garlic** and sauté it for another minute until it is fragrant. Stir in the **tomato paste**, **paprika**, and **cumin**. Cover and cook the mixture, stirring it occasionally for about 2 minutes.

2. Add the **tomatoes** and **broth** to the pot. Stir and cook the mixture for 3 minutes. Puree it with an immersion blender or standard blender until it is smooth.

3. Return the soup to the pot. Cover and simmer over low heat, about 20 minutes. Check the consistency. If the soup looks too thick, add a touch of water or more broth. Adjust the **seasoning**.

4. Add the **kale** to the soup and cook it until it is fully wilted and soft, about 5 minutes.

5. Pour the soup into bowls, garnish with **red pepper flakes** (if using), and serve.

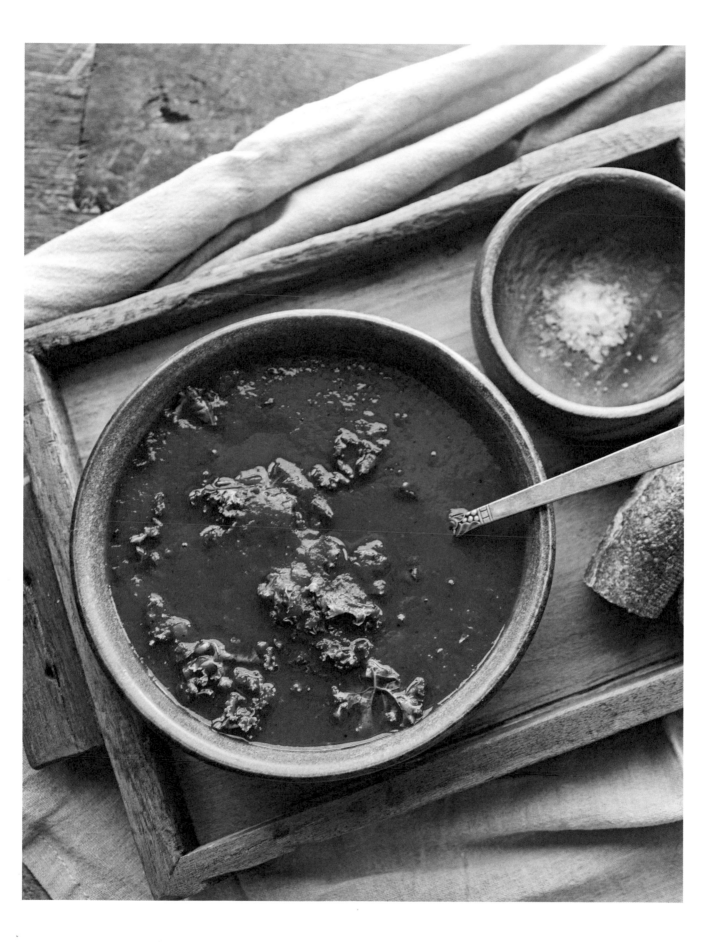

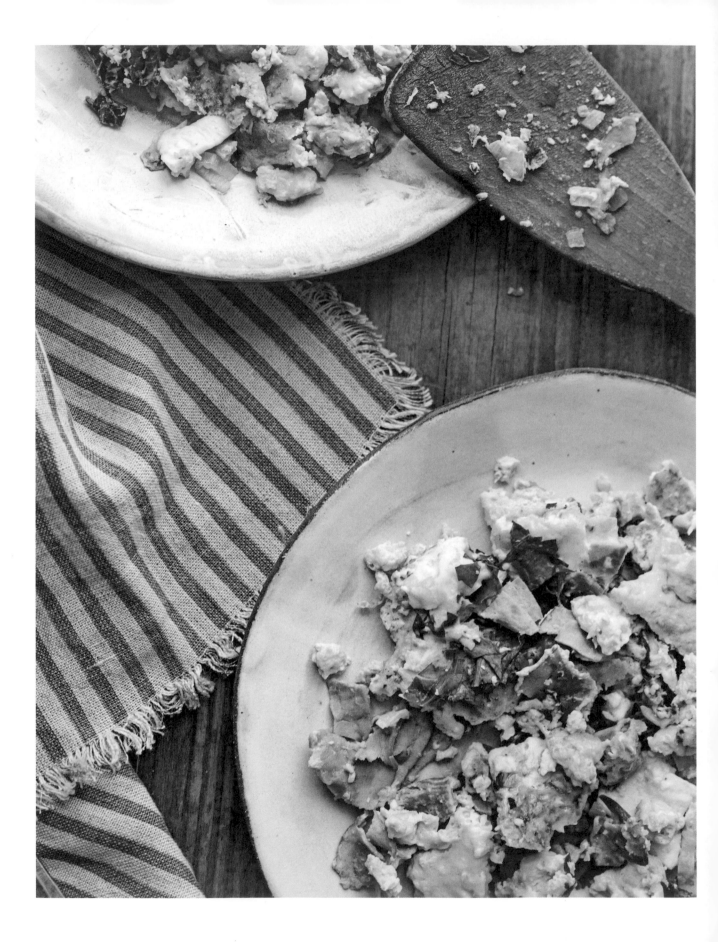

HAM, EGG, AND KALE SCRAMBLE

🕐 10 MINUTES   2 🍽   NON-VEGETARIAN 🍽️

For a hearty breakfast option, toss some fresh kale and ham into an egg scramble. If you'd like to bring more greens into your breakfast (always encouraged), double or triple the kale and go lighter on the ham.

INGREDIENTS

1 tablespoon extra virgin olive oil

1 shallot, diced

4 eggs

½ cup (4 ounces) diced ham

1 cup destemmed and ribboned kale

Pinch of pepper

DIRECTIONS

1. Heat the **olive oil** in a medium nonstick skillet over medium-high heat. Sauté the **shallot** until it is translucent, about 2 minutes.

2. Crack the **eggs** into the skillet, cover them, and let them steam over medium heat for 1 minute. Add the **ham** and cover the skillet for 2 minutes. Toss in the **kale** with some **pepper** and cover the skillet for another 2 minutes, being careful to watch the eggs so that they don't burn. Use a spatula to scramble the eggs and serve.

KIELBASA WITH ROOT VEGETABLES AND ROSEMARY

🕐 55 MINUTES   5 🍽   NON-VEGETARIAN 🍴

Roasting your favorite root vegetables, like carrots and parsnips, helps release some of their natural sugars, and in the case of carrots, it often allows some nutrients, like beta-carotene (a precursor to vitamin A) to be more bioavailable to your body. Because beta-carotene is fat-soluble, along with vitamins A, D, E, and K, adding some healthy fats like olive oil, or even a little bit of meat, to the dish will stimulate the process. But remember, a little bit of oil or meat will go a long way!

INGREDIENTS

4 small potatoes, unpeeled, scrubbed, and cut into 1 inch pieces

4 carrots, sliced

4 parsnips, sliced

2 shallots, diced

2 tablespoons extra virgin olive oil

Pinch of pepper

1 pound kielbasa

2 tablespoons rosemary leaves

DIRECTIONS

1. Preheat the oven to 400°F. Toss the **potatoes**, **carrots**, **parsnips**, and **shallots** in a bowl with the **olive oil** and **pepper**. Place the veggies on a baking pan and cover it with aluminum foil. Roast the veggies for 25 minutes, stirring them occasionally.

2. Add the **kielbasa** to the baking pan with the veggies. Sprinkle the kielbasa with **rosemary leaves**, and roast it, covered, for 15–20 minutes, or until the vegetables are tender. Transfer the kielbasa and roasted veggies to a serving bowl and toss to combine.

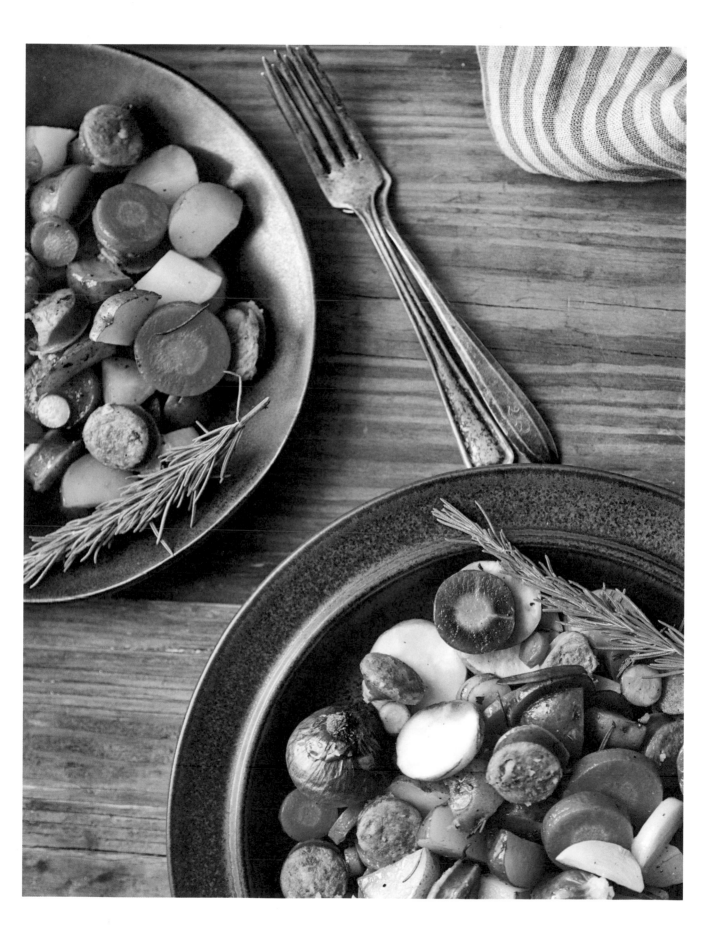

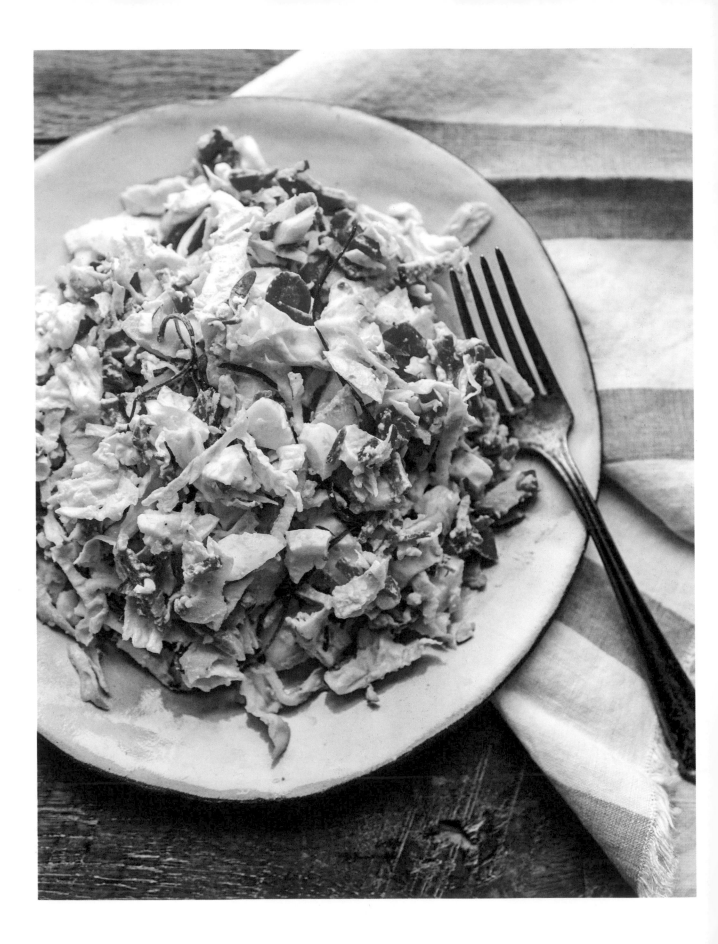

CABBAGE, EGG, AND HAM SALAD

🕐 10 MINUTES   2 🍽   NON-VEGETARIAN 🍴

This dish is like a Polish version of egg salad. Hard-boiled eggs are mashed together and combined with chopped, supple cabbage and diced ham to make a very filling meal.

INGREDIENTS

1 small head cabbage, washed and chopped

Pinch of sea salt

8 ounces ham, diced

4 eggs

½ small yellow onion, finely diced

Pinch of pepper, to taste

DIRECTIONS

1. Massage the **cabbage** with some **salt** in a bowl to soften the leaves. Add the **ham** to the bowl.

2. Hard boil the **eggs**, peel them, and chop them finely. Mix the **onion** into the eggs, then add to the cabbage mixture. Toss together. Add **pepper** to taste.

MEAL MAP 8

HAVE 15 PANTRY STAPLES READY AND SHOP FOR THESE 14 MAIN INGREDIENTS TO MAKE 7 RECIPES AND 16 SERVINGS.

RECIPES

INGREDIENTS

2 pounds mixed mushrooms

16 ounces white button mushrooms

2 leeks

2 turnips

1 bok choy

1 bunch scallions

5 beets

2 carrots

2 parsnips

2 radishes

2 medium Yukon gold potatoes

1 4-ounce package wild salmon lox

1 pound 12 ounces wild salmon fillet

2 pastured eggs

PANTRY STAPLES

Shallots × 5

Garlic × 1

Lemon × 2

Ginger × 1

Pearl barley

Salt

Pepper

Extra virgin olive oil

White wine vinegar

Balsamic vinegar

Vegetable or chicken broth

Parsley

Thyme

Bay leaves

Nutmeg

SAUCES

Tamari

Traditional Pesto

Shallot dressing

OPTIONAL

Chives

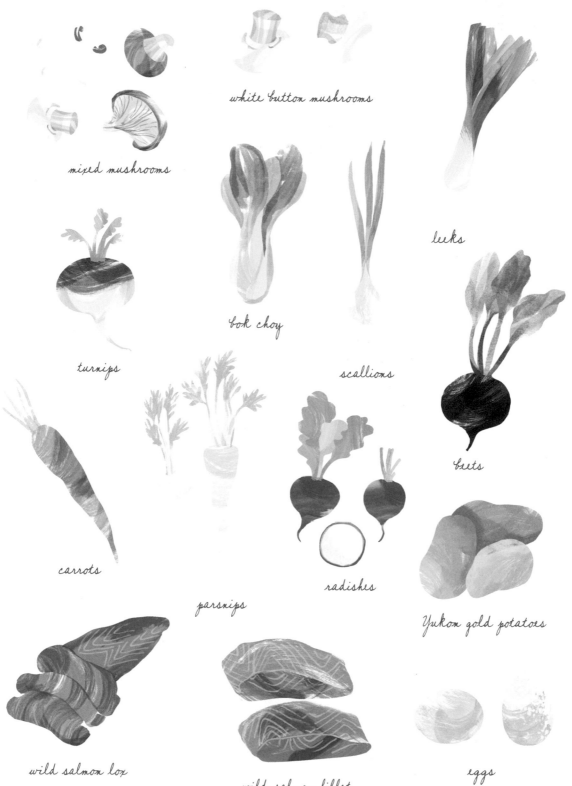

mixed mushrooms

white button mushrooms

leeks

bok choy

turnips

scallions

beets

carrots

radishes

parsnips

Yukon gold potatoes

wild salmon lox

wild salmon fillet

eggs

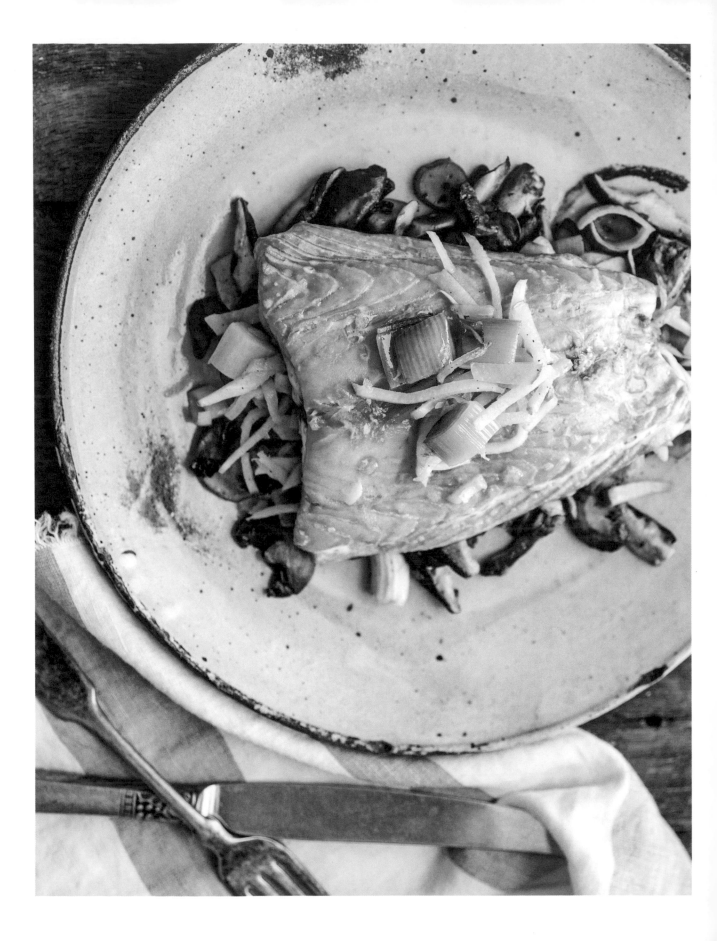

SALMON, LEEK, AND SEASONAL MUSHROOMS

🕐 15 MINUTES   2 🍲   PESCATARIAN 🐟

Wild-caught salmon has different taste, texture, and nutrition profile than farm-raised salmon, largely due to what the fish eat. Wild-caught salmon is more expensive, but worth it. Salmon offers a wealth of nutrition, from omega-3 fatty acids—an essential fat that your body needs for basic cell function—to vitamins B_{12}, B_3, B_6, and D, along with selenium, phosphorus, iodine, and choline. The combination of salmon, leeks, and mushrooms in this recipe delivers a luscious dish that just about melts in your mouth.

INGREDIENTS

½ pound mixed mushrooms, cleaned and sliced

3 tablespoons extra virgin olive oil, divided

Pinch of sea salt

Pinch of pepper

1 leek, washed, and cut into 1 inch thick slices

1 turnip, julienned

1 pound wild salmon (about 2 fillets)

DIRECTIONS

1. Lightly sauté the **mushrooms** in 1 tablespoon of the **olive oil** for about 2–3 minutes in a nonstick skillet. Season the mushrooms with **salt** and **pepper**. Transfer the mushrooms to a paper towel on a plate to absorb any excess liquid.

2. Sauté the **leeks** in the skillet with ½ tablespoon of the olive oil.

3. Add the **turnips** to the same skillet with an additional ½ tablespoon of the olive oil. Sauté the turnip for about 3 minutes. Remove the leeks and turnips from the skillet. Put them on a couple of paper towels on a plate to absorb any extra oil.

4. Place the **salmon** in a separate pan with the remaining 1 tablespoon of olive oil. Sear the fish very lightly for 7 minutes, skin-side down. Turn over the fish and sear it for another 2 minutes. Plate the wild mushrooms with a salmon fillet on top. Garnish with the leeks and turnips.

MUSHROOM RAGOUT WITH POACHED EGG

🕐 15 MINUTES   2 🍽   VEGETARIAN 🌱

Lightly sautéing mushrooms help soften their chitinous cell wall and allows you to benefit from most of the nutrients, which are many. Though nutrient and mineral density varies depending on the mushroom variety, the age and freshness of the mushrooms, and how they're grown, mushrooms are rich in copper, which helps your body make red blood cells, collagen, and connective tissue; prevent free radical build-up to protect against cancer; help with cellular metabolism and healthy brain function; and build strong bones and teeth. Plus mushrooms are super meaty, leaving you satisfied after the meal. Basically they're everything that sweets are not!

INGREDIENTS

2 tablespoons extra virgin olive oil, divided

1 pound mixed mushrooms, cleaned and sliced

Pinch of sea salt

Pinch of pepper

2 eggs

2 tablespoons white wine vinegar

3 shallots, finely diced

1 clove garlic, minced

Sprinkle of fresh chives (optional)

Sprinkle of fresh parsley (optional)

DIRECTIONS

1. Heat 1 tablespoon of the **olive oil** in a nonstick skillet and sauté the **mushrooms**. Season them with a little **salt** and **pepper**. Cover them and set them aside.

2. Poach **1 egg** in water with the **distilled vinegar** in a medium saucepan for 4 minutes. Remove the egg with a slotted spoon and place it on a paper towel on a plate. Do the same for the second egg, using the same water.

3. Heat the remaining 1 tablespoon of olive oil in a pan and sauté the **shallots** for 2 minutes or until they are translucent. Add the **garlic** and sauté for another minute until it is fragrant. Add them to the mushrooms and stir to combine.

4. Arrange the mushrooms on a serving dish, place a poached egg on top, and sprinkle with the **chives** and **parsley**.

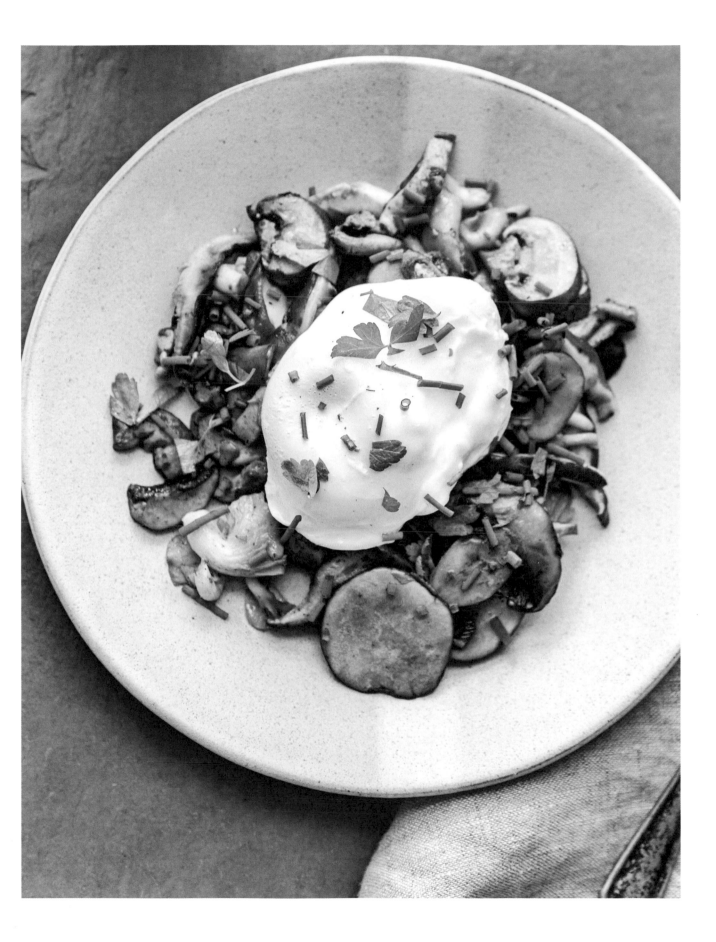

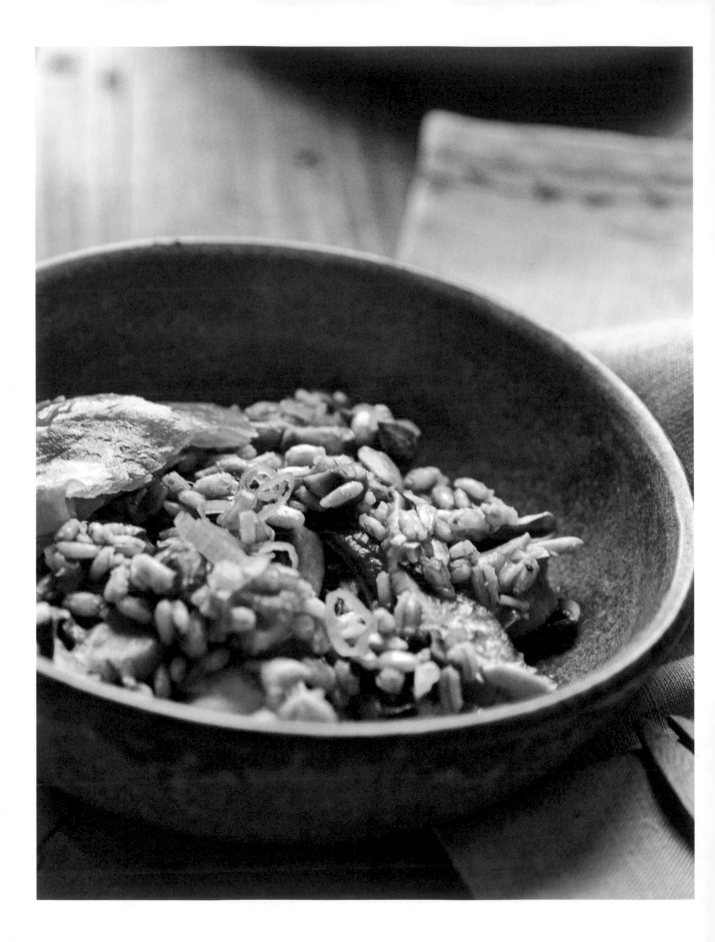

BREAKFAST BARLEY WITH LOX, MUSHROOMS, SCALLIONS, AND TAMARI

🕐 15 MINUTES   2 🍽   PESCATARIAN 🐟

If you like lox for breakfast, you can forgo the bagel and cream cheese and replace them with a risotto-like barley combined with tamari—a fermented Japanese soy sauce—savory mushrooms, and scallions. If you can find them, opt for scallion microgreens (or grow your own). I've found that young, week-old sprigs of scallions really heighten the flavor of this dish and round out the umami flavor of the mushrooms.

INGREDIENTS

1½ tablespoons extra virgin olive oil, divided

1 cup pearled barley

2½ cups mushroom or vegetable broth (see page 92 for Mushroom Broth or page 66 for Homemade Vegetable Broth)

3 scallions, thinly sliced, divided

1 shallot, finely chopped

½ pound sliced mushrooms (oyster, cremini, button, or portobello)

2 tablespoons tamari soy sauce

4 ounces wild salmon lox

DIRECTIONS

1. Add ½ tablespoon of the **olive oil** to a deep pot or pressure cooker over low heat. Add the **barley** and sauté it for 1 minute, being sure to stir so that it doesn't burn.

2. Add the **broth** and ¼ of the **scallions** to the pot. If you are using a pressure cooker, close the lid and cook the barley for 20 minutes, otherwise cook on the stovetop for 45 minutes, first by boiling for 2 minutes and then simmering for the remainder of the time. Drain the barley.

3. Heat 1 tablespoon of the olive oil over medium heat in a nonstick skillet. Add the **shallot** and sauté it for 2 minutes or until it is translucent.

4. Add the **mushrooms** to the skillet. Sauté for 3 minutes or until the mushrooms soften. When the barley is ready, stir in the mushrooms, **tamari**, and half of the scallions.

5. Serve the barley mixture in a bowl, add the **lox**, and sprinkle the remaining scallions on top.

MUSHROOM AND ROOT VEGGIE SALAD

● 60 MINUTES 2 🍽 VEGAN ✗

This is a dish that brings together the best of what's grown below ground and just above it. Root veggies like carrots, radishes, and beets add a robust flavor to juicy, roasted mushrooms. If you opt to dress the dish with pesto (the recipe is on page 44), feel free to modify it. Just clip off some of the beet greens and carrot tops and toss them into the pesto—they'll add a bit of bright, spring flavor.

INGREDIENTS

2 medium carrots, sliced thin

2 radishes, sliced thin

3 tablespoons extra virgin olive oil, divided

Pinch of sea salt

Pinch of pepper

2 beets, peeled and sliced thin

8 white button mushrooms, cleaned and sliced

Juice of 1 lemon

Sprinkle of fresh parsley

Traditional Pesto (optional; recipe on page 44)

DIRECTIONS

1. Preheat the oven to 400°F. Place the **carrots** and **radishes** in a bowl and toss them with ½ tablespoon of the **olive oil**, **salt**, and **pepper**. Arrange the carrots and radishes on a baking tray in one layer and set aside.

2. Toss the **beets** with 1 tablespoon of the olive oil, salt, and pepper, and arrange them on another baking tray. Roast the beets at 400°F for 40 minutes.

3. When the beets are halfway through their cooking time, place the other baking tray with the carrots and radishes into the oven for 20 minutes or until all the veggies are just tender. Remove and place in a covered bowl to prevent heat from escaping.

4. Toss the **mushrooms** with ½ tablespoon of the olive oil and place them in the oven on a separate baking sheet for 15 minutes at the same temperature.

5. While the mushrooms are roasting, put the remaining olive oil, **lemon juice**, parsley, salt, and pepper in a bowl and whisk them together. Plate the roasted vegetables with a drizzle of the oil and lemon juice dressing and toss them with **pesto**, if using.

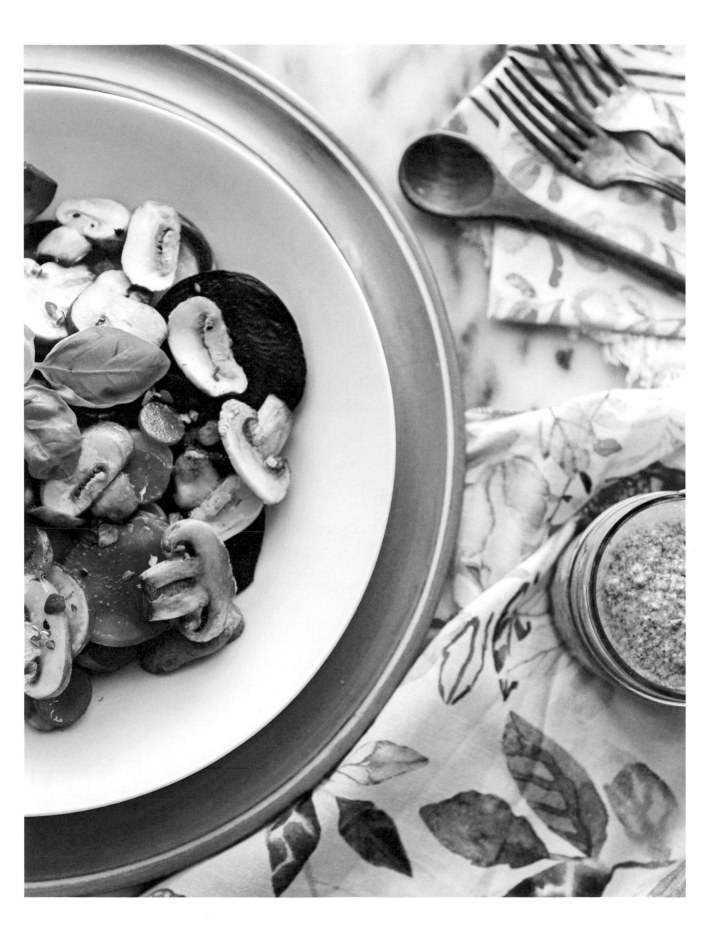

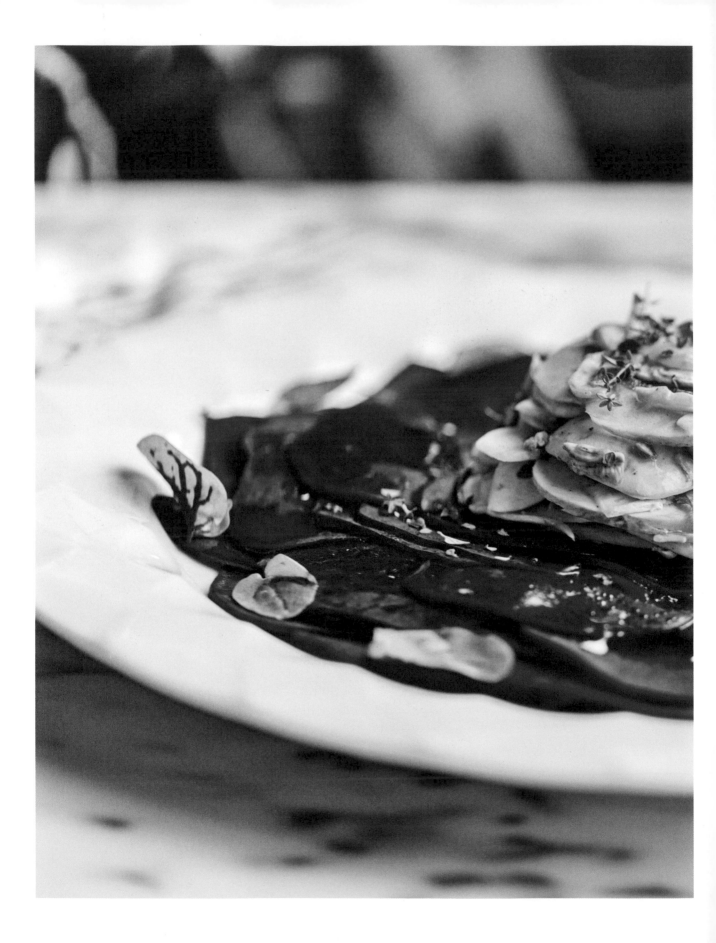

QUICK-PICKLED MUSHROOMS AND BEET CARPACCIO

60 MINUTES   2 🍽   VEGAN 🍴

Beets are quite high in sugar for a vegetable, but they are included in a sugar cleanse nonetheless, because they are chock-full of health benefits and provide a good dose of fiber. Beets are also high in folate, which is essential in making DNA and is particularly important for pregnant women, and manganese, which is essential for brain and nerve function, carbohydrate and fat metabolism, and formation of tissues and bones. The lemon juice in the recipe quickly pickles the mushrooms, adding a freshness and subtle suppleness to them, which, when combined with the thinly sliced red beets, makes for an easy-to-eat, delicious dish that can act as either an appetizer or a vegetable-centric dessert.

INGREDIENTS

3 small beets

Juice of 1 lemon, divided

1 tablespoon finely minced shallots

3 tablespoons olive oil, divided

1 tablespoon balsamic vinegar

Sea salt

Pepper

8 ounces white button mushrooms, cleaned and sliced

½ tablespoon thyme

DIRECTIONS

1. Place the small whole **beets** in a large saucepan and add **salted water**, with half of the **lemon juice**, to cover. Bring the water to a boil, reduce the heat, and simmer until the beets are tender and can be pierced with a fork, about 45 minutes. Rinse the beets until they are cool enough to handle. Remove the skins and cut the beets into thin rounds.

2. To prepare the dressing, place the **shallots** in a food processor with 2 tablespoons of the **olive oil**, plus the **vinegar**, **salt** and **pepper** to taste, and 2 tablespoons of water. Process the shallot mixture until smooth. Run the mixture through a sieve to make sure there are no remaining chunks. Set aside.

3. Place the **mushrooms** in a bowl and season them with a little salt and pepper. Add the remaining lemon juice and the remaining 1 tablespoon of the olive oil to the mushrooms, and mix them well. Let them sit for 10 minutes, mixing every couple of minutes. Add the **thyme** and stir it gently into the mushrooms.

4. Place the beets in a circle on a plate and arrange the mushroom mixture on top. Spoon the shallot dressing and any remaining mushroom juice around the plate.

TAMARI SALMON BOWL WITH SPIRALIZED PARSNIP NOODLES, ASIAN GREENS, MUSHROOMS, AND BROTH

🕐 20 MINUTES   2 🍽   PESCATARIAN 🐟

I've noticed a new restaurant trend hitting Brooklyn that's all about serving quick, healthy dishes in bowls. As a way to complement this trend I'd like to offer a quick and easy alternative. Spiralizing root veggies like parsnips and turnips (or radishes) gives an earthy sweetness and zing to this dish, while bok choy brings a refreshing bite to the umami flavors of tamari, salmon, and mushroom.

INGREDIENTS

1 medium parsnip

1 medium turnip

1 leek, washed and cut into 1 inch pieces

1½ tablespoons extra virgin olive oil, divided

2 6-ounce wild salmon fillets

2 small cloves garlic, minced

2 teaspoons ginger, minced

4 stalks bok choy

4 cups vegetable broth, store-bought, or use the recipe for Homemade Vegetable Broth on page 66

4 ounces mixed mushrooms

Pinch of sea salt

Pinch of pepper

⅓ cup scallions, chopped

DIRECTIONS

1. Spiralize the **parsnip** and **turnip** and set the "noodles" aside in a bowl.

2. Wash the **leeks** well to get rid of any gritty sand and cut the white and pale green parts into 1 inch slices. Sauté the leeks in a skillet with 1 tablespoon of the **olive oil**. Add the **salmon** and sear it for about 5 minutes on the skin side, and 3 minutes on the other side, over medium heat. Remove the skin from the fillets, discard the skin, and set the fillets aside.

3. In another skillet, add the remaining ½ tablespoon of the olive oil and the **garlic** and cook for about 1 minute over medium-high heat. Add the minced **ginger**. Cook and stir the mixture for about 1 more minute.

4. Cut off the white stems from the **bok choy**, cut the leaves into 3 to 4 inch pieces, and add them to the skillet with the garlic and ginger. Stir the mixture until the bok choy leaves have wilted a little. Add the **vegetable broth** and stir for another minute.

5 Add the **mushrooms** and the turnip and parsnip noodles to the skillet with the broth and bok choy. Season the mixture with **salt** and **pepper**, and let it cook uncovered for about 3–5 minutes or until the liquid boils for 1 minute. Right before the noodles are finished, add half of the **scallions**. Divide the noodle mixture into large bowls, place the salmon on top, and sprinkle the remainder of the scallions over the noodles and fish.

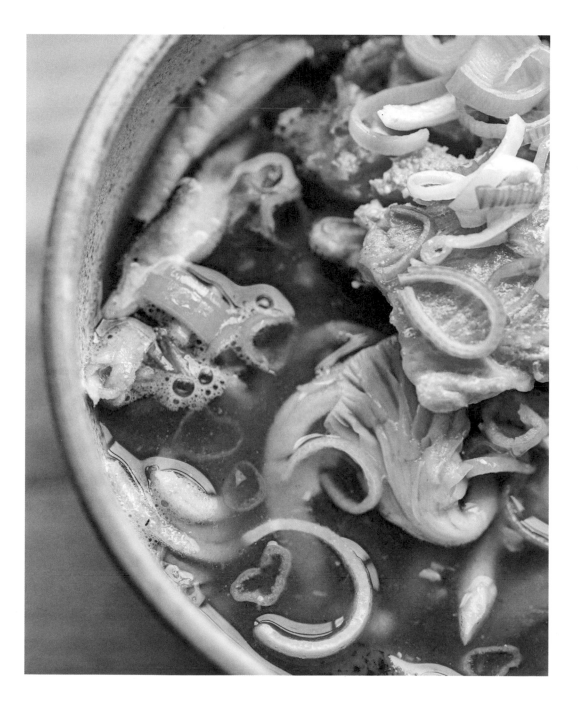

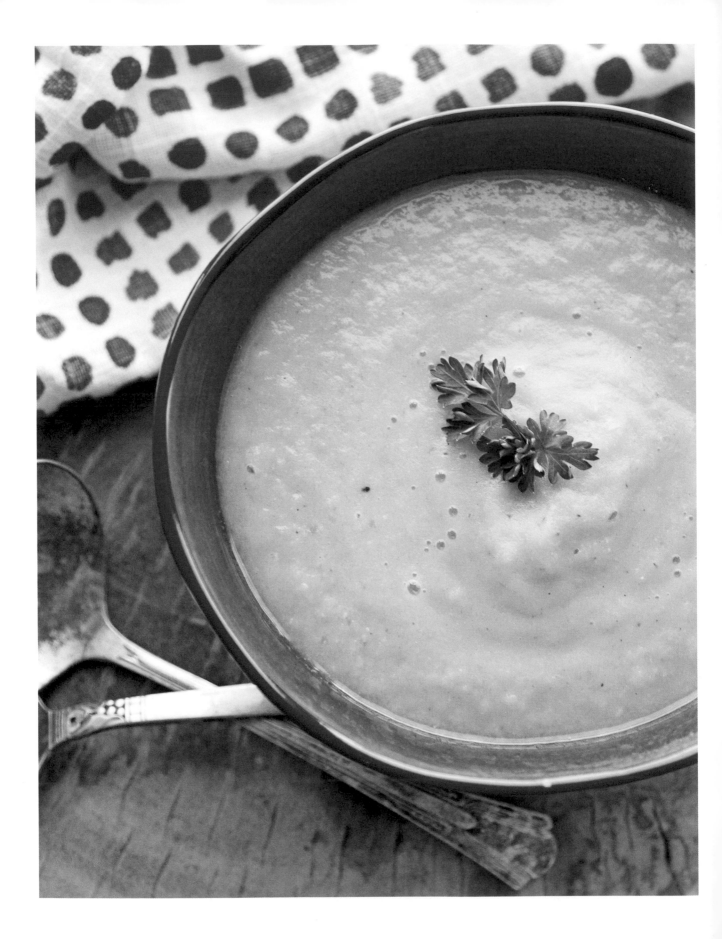

PARSNIP-POTATO PUREE SOUP

🕐 **20** MINUTES   4 🍽   VEGAN 🍴

Although I often say to leave the skins on, when you're preparing a soup with root vegetables, sometimes you want it to have a velvety mouthfeel. If that's the case, go ahead and remove the skins before sautéing the parsnips and potatoes in this luscious soup. Even without the skins, the starchiness of the two root vegetables gives the soup a rich texture that you'll want to savor slowly, spoonful by spoonful. It generally takes your brain about 20 minutes to know that you're full, so sipping your soup mindfully is a surefire way to eat less and give your brain time to catch up with your spoon!

INGREDIENTS

2 tablespoons extra virgin olive oil, divided

1 shallot, chopped

2 cloves garlic, chopped

½ pound parsnips, skins removed and diced

2 medium Yukon gold potatoes, skins removed and diced

4 cups vegetable (or chicken) broth

A couple of sprigs fresh thyme

1 bay leaf

⅛ teaspoon freshly grated or dried ground nutmeg

Pinch of sea salt, to taste

Pinch of pepper, to taste

1 teaspoon flat-leaf parsley, chopped

DIRECTIONS

1. Add 1 tablespoon of the **olive oil** to a saucepan and sauté the **shallot** for 2 minutes, or until it is translucent. Add the **garlic** and sauté it for another minute or until it is fragrant. Add the **parsnips** and **potatoes** and sauté them for another 2 minutes.

2. Add the **broth, thyme,** and **bay leaf** to the saucepan. Boil the parsnips and potatoes, partially covered, until they soften, about 15 minutes.

3. Let the soup mixture cool. Add the **nutmeg, salt,** and **pepper,** and puree the mixture with an immersion blender, or let the mixture cool and then blend it in a blender. Pour the soup into bowls and garnish it with the **parsley.**

MEAL MAP 9

Have **17** pantry staples ready and shop for these **9** main ingredients to make **6** recipes and **12** servings.

RECIPES

INGREDIENTS	PANTRY STAPLES	
5 sweet potatoes	Shallots × 5	Turmeric
9 red peppers	Garlic × 2	Cinnamon
2 bunches curly kale	Lemons × 2	Cayenne pepper
2 bunches Lacinato kale	Ginger × 1	Saffron
2 pastured eggs	Quinoa	Bay leaves
8 ounces button mushrooms	Mung beans	Cilantro
2 butternut squash	Salt	Vegetable broth
1 kabocha or delicata squash	Pepper	
2 halibut fillets	Extra virgin olive oil	
	Balsamic vinegar	

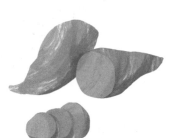

sweet potatoes

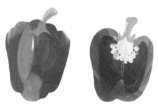

red peppers

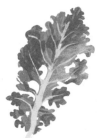

curly kale

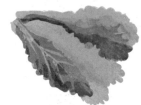

Lacinato kale

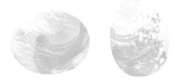

eggs

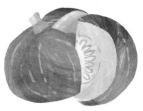

kabocha or delicata
squash

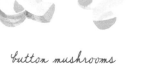

button mushrooms

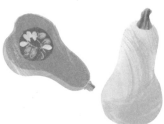

butternut squash

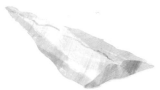

halibut fillets

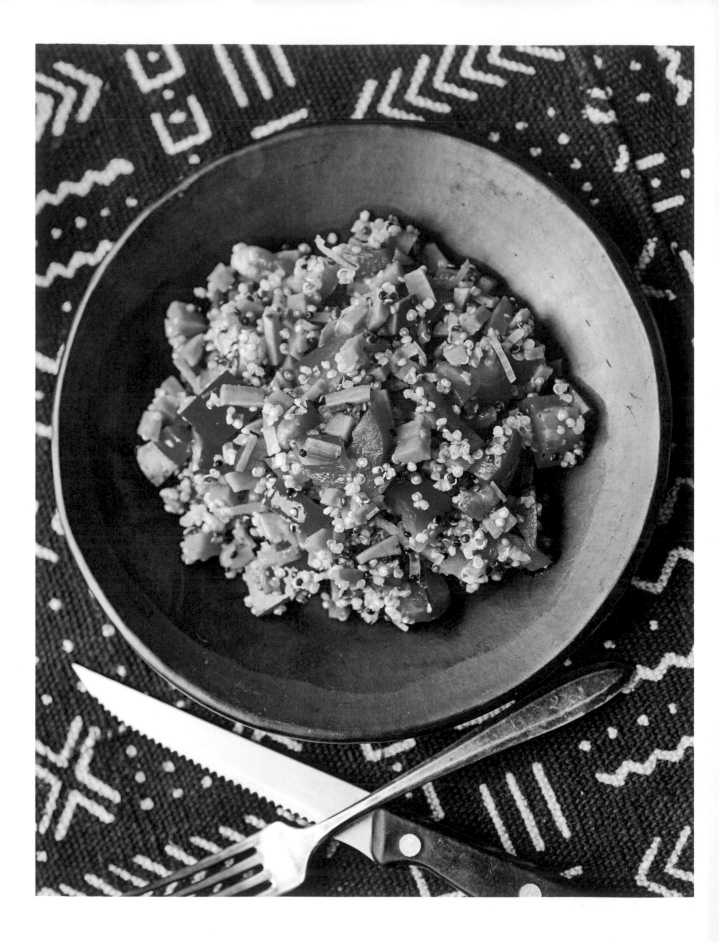

SWEET POTATO HASH OVER QUINOA AND BELL PEPPERS

⏱ 25 MINUTES   2 🍽   VEGAN ✗

Slightly sautéed red bell peppers—which are just the sweeter, more mature versions of green bell peppers that have been left to ripen on the vine—and sweet potatoes offer a natural sweetness to the rather slightly nutty yet neutral taste of quinoa. This makes a perfectly fine breakfast, lunch, or dinner.

INGREDIENTS

1 cup vegetable broth, store-bought, or use the recipe for Homemade Vegetable Broth on page 66

½ cup quinoa

2 tablespoons extra virgin olive oil

1 shallot, peeled and chopped

1 sweet potato, julienned

1 red bell pepper, stemmed, seeded, and cut in strips

Sea salt, to taste

Pepper, to taste

DIRECTIONS

1. In a medium saucepan, bring the **vegetable broth** and **quinoa** to a boil. Reduce the heat to low, cover the saucepan, and let the mixture simmer for 15–18 minutes, or until the liquid has been absorbed.

2. While the quinoa is cooking, add the **olive oil** to a nonstick skillet over medium heat. Sauté the **shallot** for 2 minutes, or until it is translucent. Add the **sweet potato** and cook it until it is tender, approximately 3–5 minutes, turning it to keep it from burning. Add the **bell pepper** and sauté it for another 2 minutes. Season the mixture with a little **salt** and **pepper**. Mix it in with the quinoa and serve.

SUNNY-SIDE UP EGG WITH KALE AND SWEET POTATO IN A RED BELL PEPPER BOAT

🕐 25 MINUTES   2 🍽   VEGETARIAN 🌿

Roasting bell peppers is one of my favorite ways to prepare them. When you roast peppers, the outer skin blisters, just like it does when you grill them. Whenever possible, look for organically produced red peppers, as pesticide residue has a tendency to stick to the skin, and if you want to eat any fruit or vegetable with the skin on, it's best to opt for an organically grown one.

INGREDIENTS

1 red pepper, stemmed, seeded, and sliced lengthwise

3 tablespoons extra virgin olive oil, divided

2 shallots, peeled and chopped

2 cups sweet potatoes, julienned

3 cups Lacinato kale, destemmed and chopped

Pinch of sea salt

Pinch of pepper

2 eggs

DIRECTIONS

1. Preheat the oven to 400°F. Place the **pepper** halves on a baking sheet, cut-side up. Roast the peppers for about 20 minutes or until they're lightly charred. Set them aside.

2. While the peppers are roasting, add 2 tablespoons of the **olive oil** to a nonstick skillet over medium heat. Sauté the **shallots** for 2 minutes, or until they're translucent. Add the **sweet potatoes** to the skillet and sauté them until they're tender, approximately 3–5 minutes, turning them so that they don't burn. Add the **kale** to the skillet and sauté it for about 2 minutes. Season the mixture with a little **salt** and **pepper**, and set it aside.

3. In a separate skillet, over medium heat, heat the remaining 1 tablespoon of olive oil over medium heat. Crack the **eggs** into the skillet. Fry the eggs for approximately 2 minutes until the whites of the eggs begin to turn opaque. Season the eggs with salt and pepper and set them aside.

4. Plate the roasted peppers. Spoon some of the sweet potato-kale mixture into each of the peppers and top them with an egg. Enjoy!

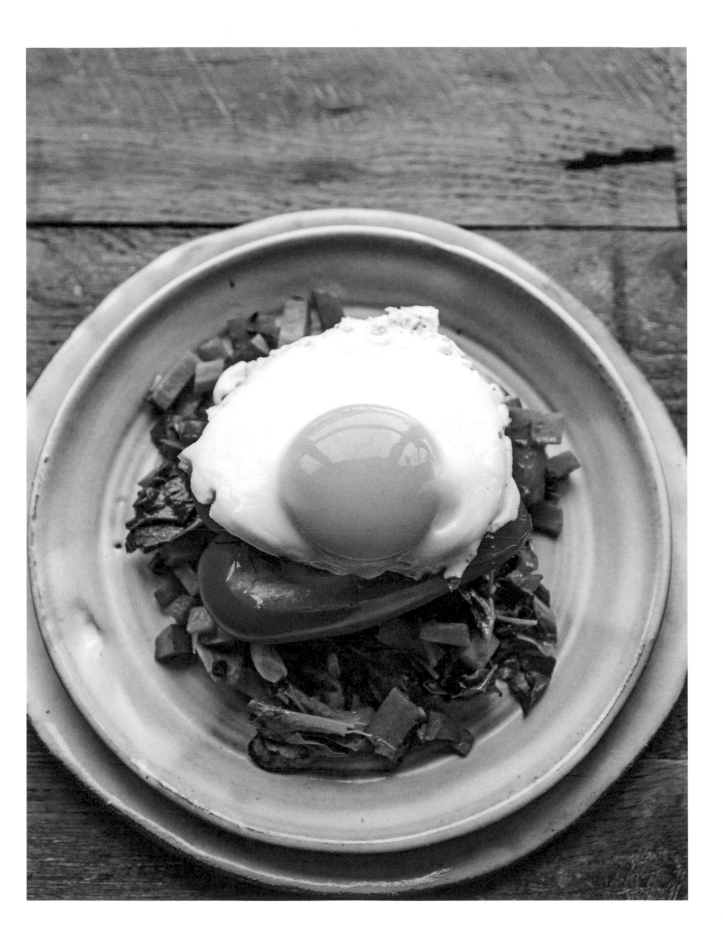

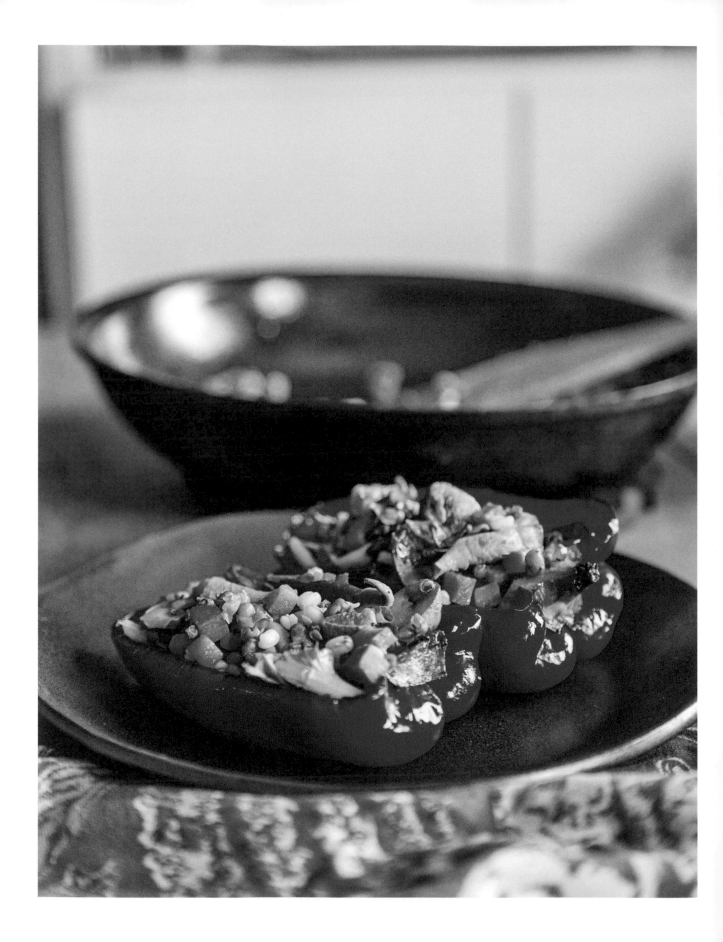

STUFFED BELL PEPPERS WITH MUNG BEANS AND VEGGIES

🕐 35 MINUTES   2 🍽   VEGAN 🍴

You may be familiar with the mung bean as a sprout, with its crisp, whitish stalk and flag-like leaf at the top. I prefer dried, sprouted mung beans, which are now easy to find in many grocery and health food stores. They are easy to prepare and can be eaten more as a meal than the fresh sprouts. Sprouting, which simply means that the seed has cracked open and a stalk has started to emerge, generally allows us to obtain more of the nutrients from the plant and digest the seed more easily. It also means that our cells and neurotransmitters will function more efficiently.

INGREDIENTS

½ cup mung beans, sorted

½ cup cubed sweet potato

3½ tablespoons extra virgin olive oil, divided

2 cloves garlic, minced, divided

2 red bell peppers, halved, stemmed, and seeded

Pinch of sea salt

Pinch of pepper

½ cup white button mushrooms, sliced

2 cups Lacinato kale, washed, deveined, and chopped

1 tablespoon lemon juice

DIRECTIONS

1. Pour 1½ cups of **water** into a medium saucepan and add the **mung beans**. Bring the water to a boil and then let it simmer, uncovered, for 25 minutes. (If sprouted, simmer for an extra 5 minutes.)

2. While the water is simmering, preheat the oven to 400°F. Toss the **sweet potato** with 1 tablespoon of the **olive oil** and half of the minced **garlic** in a large bowl. Season with **salt** and **black pepper**, and arrange the sweet potato on a baking sheet. Roast for about 25 minutes.

3. Lightly brush the **peppers** with 1 tablespoon of the olive oil, and sprinkle them with salt and pepper. Place the peppers, cut-side down, on another baking sheet. Bake the peppers until they are just tender, around 15 minutes. Let them cool slightly, then turn them cut-side up.

4. Add ½ tablespoon of olive oil to a nonstick skillet and sauté the **mushrooms** over medium heat for 1 minute. Massage the **kale** with the remaining 1 tablespoon of olive oil and **lemon juice** and add it to the mushrooms in the skillet. Cover the skillet and let the kale steam for about 1 minute. Remove the mushrooms and kale from the skillet and toss them in a bowl with the mung beans and the sweet potato. Spoon mixture into peppers.

STEWED WINTER SQUASH, SWEET POTATO, AND RED BELL PEPPER SOUP

🕐 25 MINUTES   2 🍽   VEGAN 🍴

INGREDIENTS

1 tablespoon extra virgin olive oil

2 large shallots, finely chopped

3 garlic cloves, finely chopped

2 teaspoons ground ginger

2 teaspoons ground turmeric

1 cinnamon stick (or 1 teaspoon of cinnamon)

Pinch of cayenne pepper

4 cups vegetable broth, store-bought, or use the recipe for Homemade Vegetable Broth on page 66

⅛ teaspoon ground saffron threads

1 bay leaf

2 cups peeled and cubed butternut squash

2 cups peeled and cubed kabocha or delicata squash

1 cup peeled and cubed sweet potato

¼ teaspoon sea salt

Pinch of pepper, to taste

1 cup seeded and chopped red bell pepper

Sprinkle of cilantro leaves

This sweetly spiced soup brings to mind a cool autumn day. It is richly flavored with warming spices like ginger, turmeric, cinnamon, and cayenne, and sweetened with winter squash, sweet potatoes, and red bell pepper.

DIRECTIONS

1. Add the **olive oil** to a deep pot over low heat and sauté the **shallots** for 2 minutes or until they are translucent. Add the **garlic**, **ginger**, **turmeric**, **cinnamon**, and **cayenne pepper**. Stir the mixture over low heat for 1–2 minutes.

2. Pour in the **broth** and add the **saffron** to the pot. Increase the heat to medium and bring the broth to a boil.

3. Add the **bay leaf**, **butternut squash**, **kabocha** or **delicata squash**, **sweet potato**, and a pinch of **salt** and freshly ground black pepper to the pot. Cover and simmer for 10 more minutes.

4. Add the **red bell pepper** to the pot and simmer the mixture for another 5 minutes, until the vegetables are tender. Remove the cinnamon stick and bay leaf. Transfer the soup to a bowl and scatter **cilantro leaves** over the top.

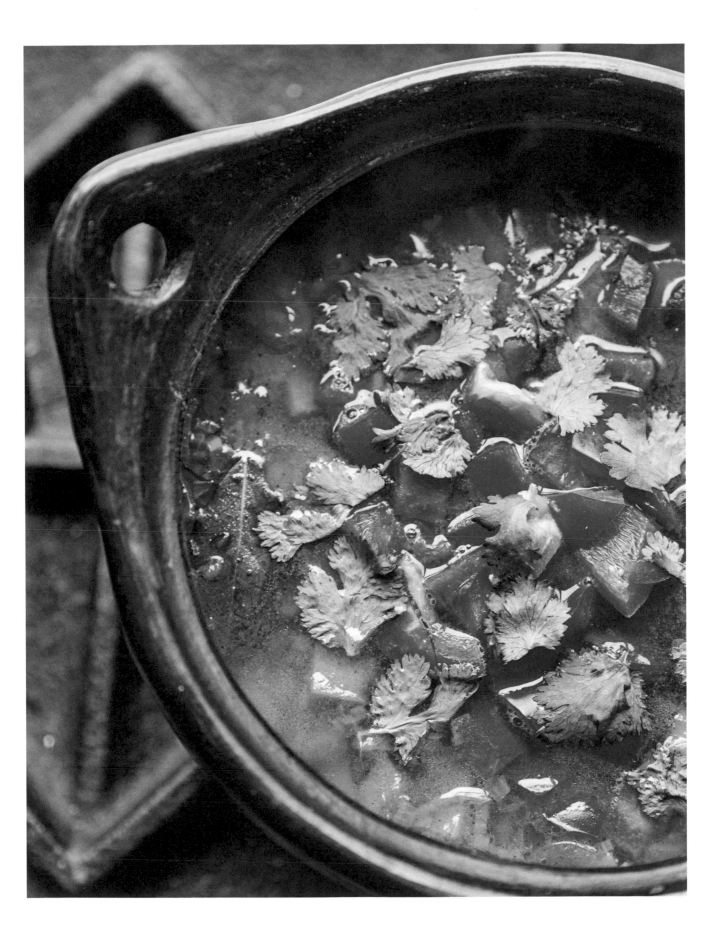

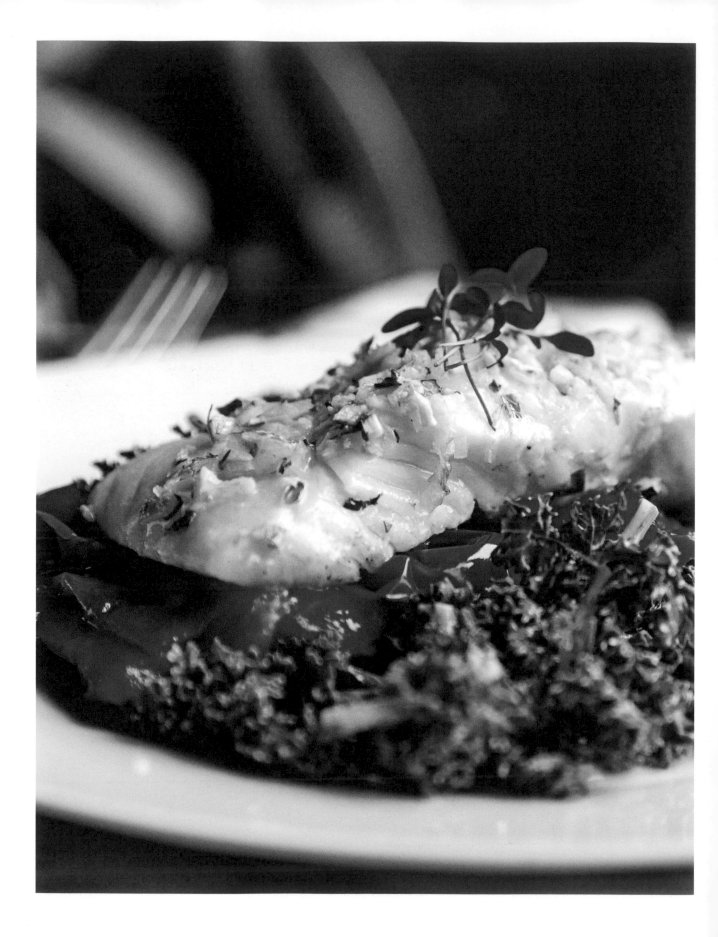

MARINATED HALIBUT WITH ROASTED RED BELL PEPPERS AND KALE

● 60 MINUTES   2 🍽   PESCATARIAN 🐟

Halibut is an easy fish to like. It's relatively mild, flakes nicely, and takes on flavor well. It is high in protein, potassium, selenium, vitamins B_{12} and B_6, and omega-3 fatty acids. Buy Pacific-caught halibut, if you can, as Atlantic halibut are becoming rare and are bottom trawled, which is severely damaging to the ocean ecosystem. Halibut raised in aquaculture is decent, but not as good for the environment or your health as wild-caught fish.

INGREDIENTS

2 red bell peppers

3 tablespoons extra virgin olive oil, divided

Pinch of sea salt

Pinch of pepper

½ tablespoon lemon zest

2 tablespoons lemon juice

1 tablespoon balsamic vinegar

2 garlic cloves, minced

2 halibut fillets

4 cups curly kale, destemmed and chopped

DIRECTIONS

1. Preheat the oven to 400°F. Place the **bell peppers** on a parchment-lined baking sheet. Lightly brush them with 1 tablespoon of the **olive oil**, sprinkle with **salt** and **pepper**, and roast them until they are soft and the skins have split, around 30 minutes. Transfer the bell peppers to a bowl and cover them with plastic wrap. Let them steam.

2. When the bell peppers are cool, peel them, slice them in half lengthwise, and remove the stem and seeds. Cut the peppers into strips and place them in a bowl.

3. In a small bowl, mix the **lemon zest**, **lemon juice**, **balsamic vinegar**, **garlic**, **salt**, **pepper**, and 1 tablespoon of the olive oil. Marinate the **halibut fillets**, skin-side down, in a glass baking dish for at least 15 minutes, but more if you have the time. Place the halibut in the oven and cook for 12–15 minutes at 400°F, or until the fish flakes with a fork.

4. Massage the **kale** with the remaining 1 tablespoon of olive oil and a pinch of salt and pepper. Wilt the kale in a nonstick skillet over medium heat for about 1 minute. Plate the kale and bell pepper and top with a halibut fillet.

STUFFED SWEET BELL PEPPERS WITH QUINOA AND SQUASH

🕐 **35** MINUTES   2 🍽   VEGAN 🍴

Foods that double as edible bowls, like halved sweet bell peppers, score high on my good food list, since there is no waste! Buy bell peppers from your local farmers market, if you can, since the skin on non-organic store-bought peppers are sometimes covered with pesticide residues and wax. If you must use store-bought peppers, gently clean the outsides with a natural veggie wash, which you can make from a squeeze of lemon, a dash of distilled vinegar, and clean water.

INGREDIENTS

1 cup vegetable broth, store-bought, or use the recipe for Homemade Vegetable Broth on page 66

½ cup quinoa

1 cup peeled and cubed butternut squash

2 tablespoons extra virgin olive oil, divided

2 cloves garlic, minced, divided

Pinch of sea salt

Pinch of pepper

2 small red bell peppers, halved, stemmed, and seeded

DIRECTIONS

1. In a medium saucepan, bring the **vegetable broth** and **quinoa** to a boil. Reduce the heat to low and let the broth simmer, covered, for 15–18 minutes, or until all the liquid has been absorbed. Set the saucepan aside with the cover on.

2. While the quinoa is being prepared, preheat the oven to 400°F. Toss the **butternut squash** with 1 tablespoon of the **olive oil** and half of the minced **garlic** in a large bowl. Season the squash with **salt** and **black pepper**. Arrange the squash on a parchment-lined baking sheet. Roast the squash until it is tender, about 25 minutes.

3. Lightly brush the **red bell peppers** with the remaining 1 tablespoon of olive oil and remaining garlic and place them in a large bowl. Season the peppers with salt and black pepper and place them, cut-side down, on another baking sheet. Bake the peppers until they are just tender, 10–15 minutes. Let the peppers cool slightly. Turn them cut-side up.

4. When the peppers are cool, combine the quinoa and squash. Fill the bell peppers with the mixture and serve.

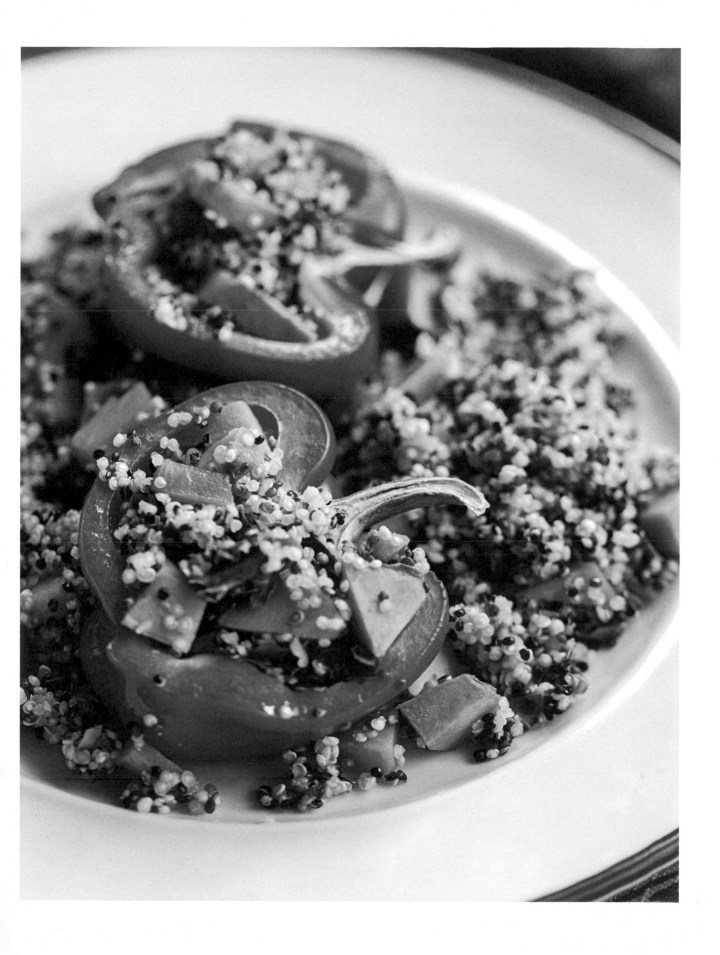

MEAL MAP 10

Have **18** pantry staples ready and shop for these **15** main ingredients to make **8** recipes and **16** servings.

RECIPES

INGREDIENTS
8 pastured eggs

3 spaghetti squash

2 bunches scallions

1 green pepper

1 red bell pepper

1 small banana

4 jalapeño peppers

2 cups enoki mushrooms

8 ounces oyster mushrooms

2 bunches kale

4 13.5-ounce cans coconut milk

1¼ pounds shell-on medium shrimp

1 cup mustard microgreens

¾ cup dried wakame seaweed

1 green apple

PANTRY STAPLES
Shallots × 4

Ginger × 3

Garlic × 2

Red onions × 1

Limes × 4

Vegetable or chicken broth

Mung beans

Extra virgin olive oil

Apple cider vinegar

Sea salt

Pepper

Almond flour

Coconut flour

Coconut oil

Sesame oil

Lemongrass

Cilantro

OPTIONAL
Scallion microgreens

Sesame seeds

Kefir

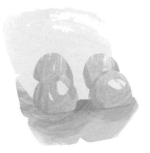

eggs

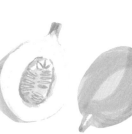

spaghetti squash

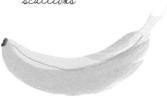

green apple

scallions

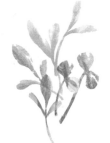

mustard microgreens

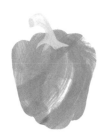

green pepper

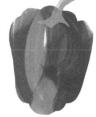

red bell pepper

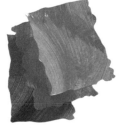

banana

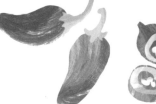

jalapeño peppers

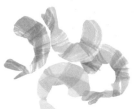

dried wakame seaweed

enoki mushrooms

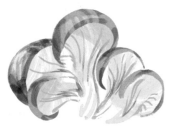

oyster mushrooms

wild-caught shrimp

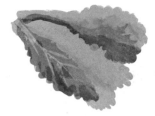

kale

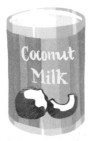

coconut milk

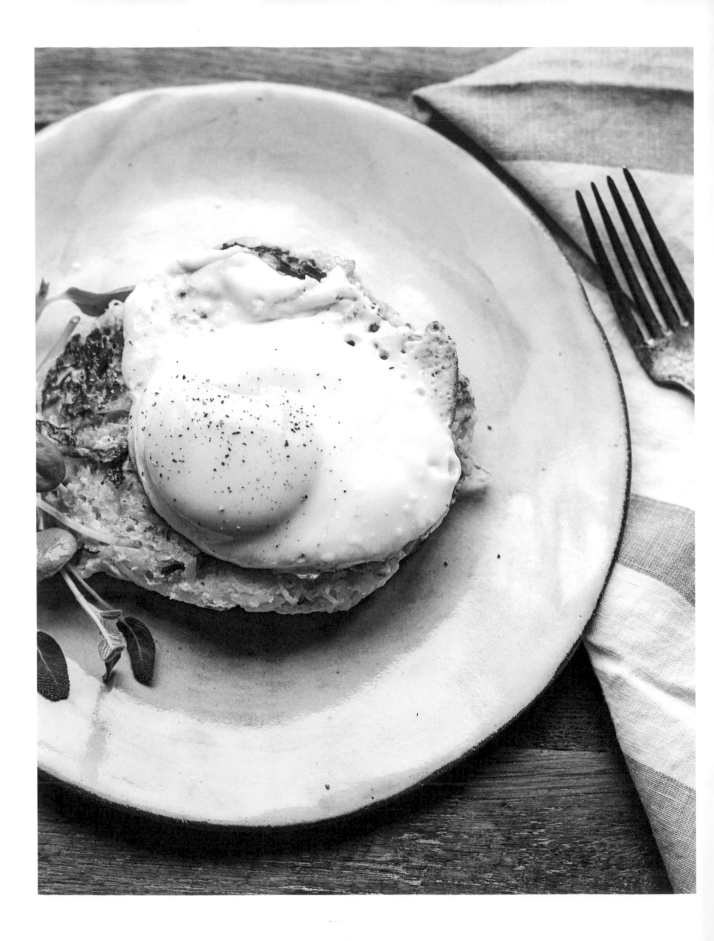

SPAGHETTI SQUASH–SCALLION PATTIES WITH A SUNNY-SIDE UP EGG

🕐 45 MINUTES   2 🍽   VEGETARIAN 🌱

Some real magic happens when you roast this gourd: the canary-yellow flesh of the spaghetti squash pulls away in strands that look similar to—you guessed it—spaghetti! And you can easily prepare it in advance, since roasting does take a while. Just scoop out the flesh you're not immediately using and keep it in a sealed container in the fridge. Spaghetti squash mixed with a little egg browns up really nicely in the skillet, making it easy to make either delicious patties or hash browns!

INGREDIENTS

2 tablespoons extra virgin olive oil, divided

½ medium spaghetti squash, deseeded

Pinch of sea salt

Pinch of pepper

3 eggs

2 tablespoons finely chopped scallions, divided

1 shallot, finely diced

DIRECTIONS

NOTE: *Prepare the squash the day before so that it's ready to go for breakfast.*

1. Preheat the oven to 375°F. Brush the inside of the **spaghetti squash** with 1 tablespoon of the **olive oil** and sprinkle with **sea salt** and **freshly ground black pepper**. Place the cut side of the squash facedown in a glass baking dish and bake for about 40 minutes, or until you can easily pierce the squash with a fork. Scrape the flesh out in long strands using a fork. Spread the strands on paper towels to absorb any excess moisture.

2. Crack **1 egg** into a large bowl and give it a good stir. Add 1 tablespoon of the **scallions** to the mixture. Add the cooked squash to the bowl and mix well.

3. Press the squash mixture between your palms to form about four little patties. Heat 1 tablespoon of the olive oil in a nonstick skillet over medium heat. Gently place the patties in the warmed skillet and let them cook for 5–7 minutes per side or until they start to brown. Transfer the patties to paper towels to drain off any excess oil.

4. Once the scallion patties are removed from the skillet, add the remaining 1 tablespoon of olive oil. Sauté the **shallot** for 2 minutes or until it's translucent. Crack the remaining eggs into the skillet. Cover the skillet and let the eggs "steam" on medium for about 1 minute or until the white is opaque and the outside of the yolk has set. Sprinkle the eggs with a little salt and pepper. Use a metal spatula to carefully remove the eggs. Plate the patties and eggs and sprinkle with the remaining 1 tablespoon of scallions.

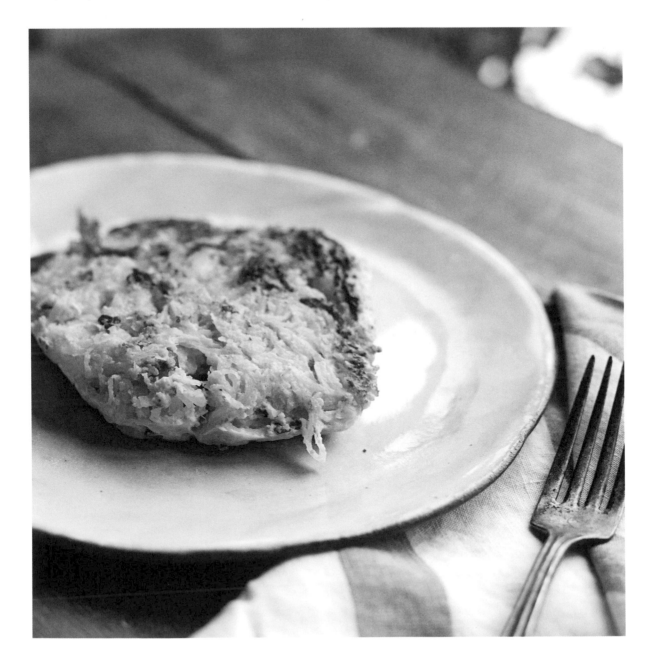

LEMONGRASS SPAGHETTI SQUASH SHRIMP SOUP

● 🕐 80 MINUTES   2 🍽   PESCATARIAN 🐟

Spaghetti squash is a fun and tasty substitute for noodles, particularly in soups. The flesh of the spaghetti squash has a mildly sweet flavor that perfectly complements the savory elements in this soul-comforting soup.

INGREDIENTS

½ medium spaghetti squash, deseeded

3 tablespoons extra virgin olive oil

Pinch of sea salt, to taste

Pinch of freshly ground black pepper, to taste

¾ pound shell-on medium shrimp

4 scallions, thinly sliced

1 lemongrass stalk, tough outer layers removed, thinly sliced

1 2-inch piece ginger, peeled and thinly sliced

3 garlic cloves, thinly sliced

4 cups vegetable or chicken broth, store-bought, or use the recipe for Homemade Vegetable Broth on page 66 or Homemade Chicken Broth on page 78

2 tablespoons cilantro sprigs

2 teaspoons minced jalapeño peppers

2 lime wedges

½ teaspoon toasted sesame seeds (optional)

2 tablespoons scallion microgreens (optional garnish)

DIRECTIONS

NOTE: *Prepare the squash the day before so that it's ready to go.*

1. Preheat the oven to 375°F. Brush the inside of the **spaghetti squash** with 1 tablespoon of the **olive oil** and sprinkle the squash with **salt** and **pepper**. Place the cut side facedown in a glass baking dish and bake for about 40 minutes, or until you can easily pierce the squash with a fork. Scrape the flesh out in long strands using a fork. Spread the strands on paper towels to absorb any excess moisture.

2. Meanwhile, peel and devein the **shrimp**, if needed. Place the shrimp in a medium-size bowl; cover and chill until you are ready to use them.

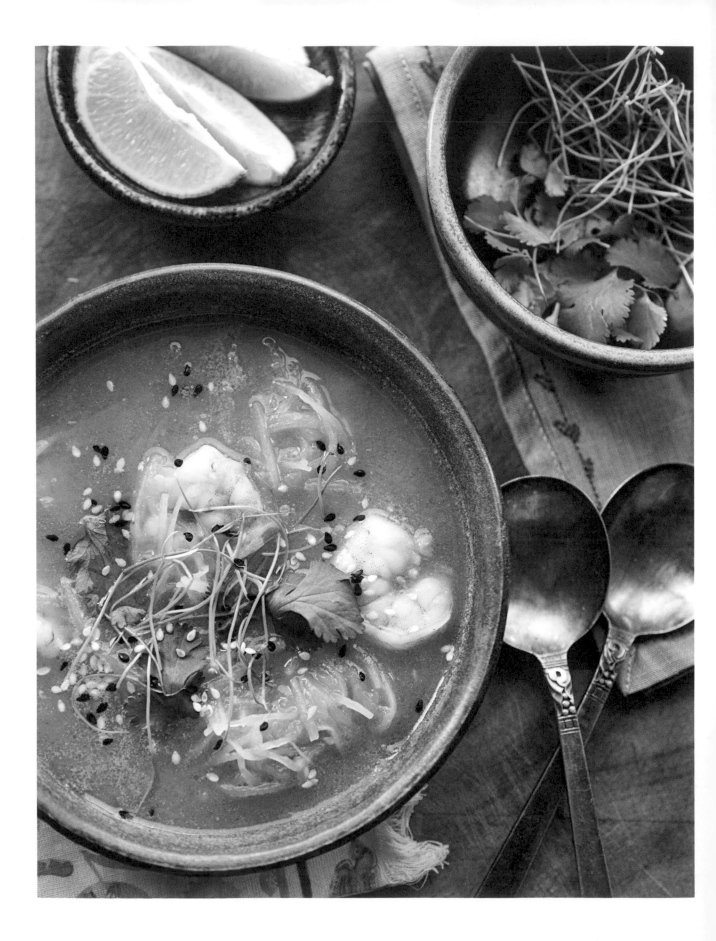

3. Heat the remaining 2 tablespoons of olive oil in a deep pot over medium heat and add the **scallions**, **lemongrass**, **ginger**, and **garlic**. Reduce the heat to low, and cook the mixture, stirring it occasionally, until it has softened, about 2 minutes. Add the **broth** and bring it to a boil. Reduce the heat and simmer the mixture until the flavors marry and come together, about 30 minutes. Strain the mixture through a fine-mesh sieve into a clean medium-size saucepan.

4. Bring the broth to a boil. Reduce the heat, add the chilled shrimp, and simmer the broth until the shrimp are cooked through, about 2 minutes; season with salt.

5. Divide the squash among bowls and ladle the shrimp and broth over it. Top the soup with the **cilantro** and **jalapeño peppers** and serve with **lime wedges** to squeeze over the soup. If you have **toasted sesame seeds** and **scallion microgreens** on hand, use them as a garnish for the soup.

SPAGHETTI SQUASH NOODLE, SPROUTED MUNG BEAN, AND ENOKI MUSHROOM SOUP

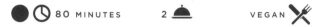

● 🕐 80 MINUTES   2 🍽   VEGAN ✕

I love soups that have a multitude of textures, and this soup is no exception. Squash noodles, beans, mushrooms, and greens stand out on their own in this soup, and yet mingle together as well.

INGREDIENTS

½ spaghetti squash

3 tablespoons extra virgin olive oil, divided

Salt and pepper

1 shallot, diced

1 garlic clove, diced

¼ cup pureed ginger

1½ 13.5-ounce cans coconut milk

3 cups vegetable broth, divided, store-bought, or use the recipe for Homemade Vegetable Broth on page 66

½ cup mung beans, sprouted

2 cups enoki mushrooms

1 cup mustard microgreens

DIRECTIONS

NOTE: *Prepare the squash the day before so that it's ready to go.*

1. Preheat the oven to 375°F. Brush the inside of the **spaghetti squash** half with 1 tablespoon of the **olive oil** and sprinkle with **sea salt** and **freshly ground black pepper**. Place the cut side facedown in a glass baking dish and bake for about 40 minutes, or until you can easily pierce the squash with a fork. Scrape the flesh out in long strands using a fork. Spread the strands on paper towels to absorb any excess moisture.

2. Heat the remaining 2 tablespoons of olive oil in a deep pot over medium heat and sauté the **shallot** for 2 minutes, or until it's translucent. Add the **garlic** and **ginger** and sauté them for another minute. Pour in the **coconut milk** and half of the **vegetable broth**. Bring it to a boil, and then reduce the heat and simmer the broth until the flavors marry and come together, about 30 minutes. Strain the broth through a fine-mesh sieve into a clean medium saucepan.

3. While the coconut milk-broth mixture is cooking, in a separate saucepan, combine the **mung beans** with the remaining vegetable broth and cook for 18 minutes.

4. Combine the two broth mixtures. Add the **mushrooms** to the broth and let it simmer, covered, for another 2–3 minutes.

5. Divide the squash among bowls, ladle the soup over it, and top with fresh **mustard microgreens** and a pinch of salt and pepper to taste.

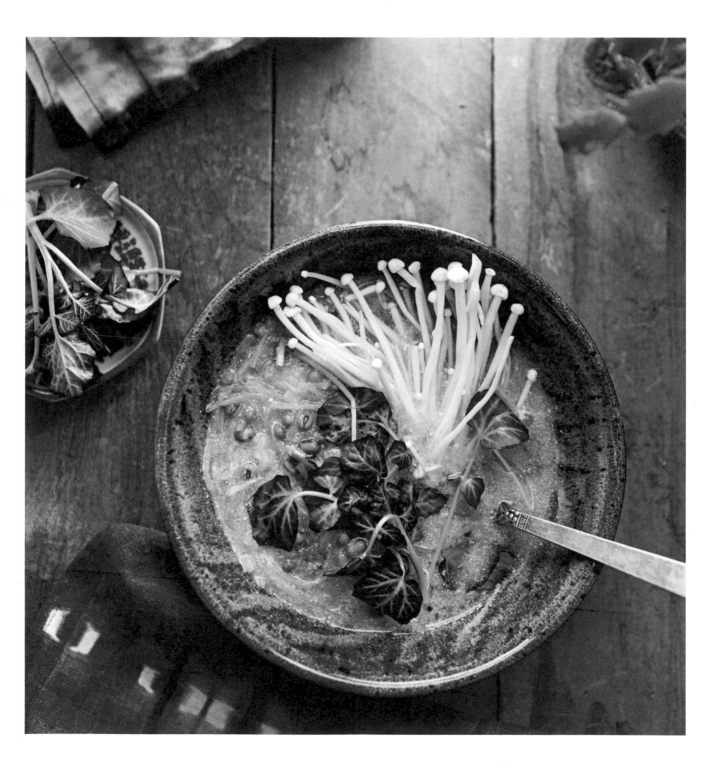

MUSHROOM CEVICHE

🕐 **20 MINUTES**   🍽 **2**   **VEGAN** ✖️
(BEST IF SITS OVERNIGHT)

I loved the mushroom ceviche that was served at a vegan restaurant that opened and then closed all too quickly on my street. I never got their recipe for ceviche, but, remembering the taste notes like an old song, I think I got as close to the original as you can get.

INGREDIENTS

2 garlic cloves

8 ounces oyster mushrooms, sliced thin

1 small red onion, sliced thin

½ green bell pepper, julienned

½ red bell pepper, julienned

1 teaspoon finely chopped jalapeño

¼ cup freshly squeezed lime juice

2 tablespoons apple cider vinegar

½ teaspoon ginger juice, store-bought or homemade

1 tablespoon toasted sesame oil

¼ teaspoon sea salt

⅛ teaspoon black pepper

1 tablespoon chopped cilantro

¼ cup dry wakame seaweed

DIRECTIONS

1. In a nonstick skillet, roast the **garlic** cloves until they are brown on all sides. Mash the garlic and place it in a large bowl with the **mushrooms**, **onion**, **red** and **green bell peppers**, and **jalapeño**. Stir to combine.

2. In a separate bowl, whisk together the **lime juice**, **vinegar**, **ginger juice**, **sesame oil**, **salt**, **pepper**, and **cilantro**. (To make ginger juice, squeeze minced ginger through a nutbag or cheesecloth until juice is released.)

3. Put the **dry seaweed** in a third small bowl and fill it with cold water. If you like your seaweed crunchy, soak it for 5 minutes; if you like it tender, soak it for 10 minutes.

4. Drain the seaweed and squeeze out any excess water. Add the seaweed to the mushroom mixture. Pour the lime juice mixture over it and let it sit overnight.

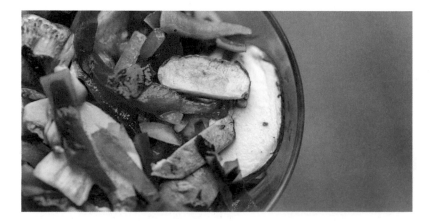

GINGERED KALE, GREEN APPLE, AND SEAWEED SALAD

🕐 15 MINUTES   🍽 2   VEGAN 🍴

Diets high in sugar cause inflammation in the system. Sea vegetables, as they are called, are loaded with health benefits, offering a wide range of mineral content that are particularly good at fighting inflammation. Luckily, seaweed is becoming more available to home cooks, particularly wakame, which you may recognize as one of the principal ingredients in miso soup.

INGREDIENTS

½ green apple, matchsticked

½ cup dried wakame seaweed

2 tablespoons sesame oil

1 tablespoon peeled and minced ginger

1 bunch kale, washed, destemmed, and chopped

Toasted sesame seeds (optional)

DIRECTIONS

1. Matchstick **apple** and set aside.

2. Put the **seaweed** in a small bowl and fill it with cold water. If you like your seaweed crunchy, soak it for 5 minutes; if you like it tender, soak it for 10 minutes. Drain the seaweed and squeeze out any excess water. Add 1 teaspoon of the **sesame oil** and the **ginger**.

3. Heat the remaining 1 tablespoon of sesame oil in nonstick skillet over medium heat. Add the chopped **kale**. Gently mix the kale in the skillet in order to coat it with the oil and lower the heat. Cook the kale for about 3 minutes, until it is wilted.

4. Mix the kale and apples into the seaweed ginger mixture, and garnish with toasted **sesame seeds**, if you like.

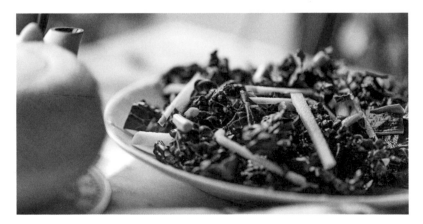

COCONUT AND LEMONGRASS SHRIMP SOUP WITH CRISPY GINGERED KALE

🕐 50 MINUTES   2 🍽   PESCATARIAN 🐟

INGREDIENTS

½ spaghetti squash

4 tablespoons extra virgin olive oil

Sea salt

Freshly ground black pepper

½ pound fresh shell-on medium shrimp, cleaned and deveined

2 tablespoons chopped scallions

1 lemongrass stalk, tough outer layers removed, thinly sliced

1 shallot, diced

1 garlic clove, diced

1 teaspoon finely diced jalapeño, plus more for garnish

¼ cup pureed ginger, divided for use

1½ 13.5-ounce cans coconut milk

2 cups vegetable broth, store-bought, or use the recipe for Homemade Vegetable Broth on page 66

½ bunch kale

2 tablespoons chopped cilantro

There's something enriching and comforting about a bowl of coconut milk infused with the flavor of lemongrass. It transports us simultaneously to a tropical island and also to the warmth of our mother's arms.

DIRECTIONS

NOTE: *Prepare the squash the day before so that it's ready to go.*

1. Preheat the oven to 375°F. Brush the inside of the **spaghetti squash** with 1 tablespoon of the **olive oil** and sprinkle with **sea salt** and **freshly ground black pepper**. Place the cut side of the squash facedown in a glass baking dish and bake for about 40 minutes, or until you can easily pierce the squash with a fork. Scrape the flesh out in long strands using a fork. Spread the strands on paper towels to absorb any excess moisture.

2. Place the **shrimp** in a medium-size bowl; cover and chill the shrimp until you are ready to use them.

3. Heat 2 tablespoons of the olive oil in a deep pot over medium heat and add the **scallions, shallot, lemongrass, garlic, jalapeño**, and 3 tablespoons of **ginger puree**. Reduce the heat to low and cook, stirring it occasionally, until the vegetables have softened, about 2 minutes. Add the **coconut milk** and **broth** and bring it to a boil. Reduce the heat and simmer the broth until the flavors marry and come together, about 30 minutes. Strain the broth through a fine-mesh sieve into a clean medium saucepan.

4. While the flavors are setting in the broth, rub the **kale** with 1 tablespoon of the olive oil and the remaining ginger. Bake the kale on a baking sheet for 10 minutes at 375°F. Set it aside.

5. Bring the broth to a boil. Reduce the heat, add the chilled shrimp, and simmer the broth until the shrimp are cooked through, about 2 minutes. Season the broth with salt, and add half of the chopped **cilantro**.

6. Divide the squash among bowls and ladle the shrimp and broth over it. Top the soup with the remaining cilantro, extra jalapeño peppers, and the crispy kale.

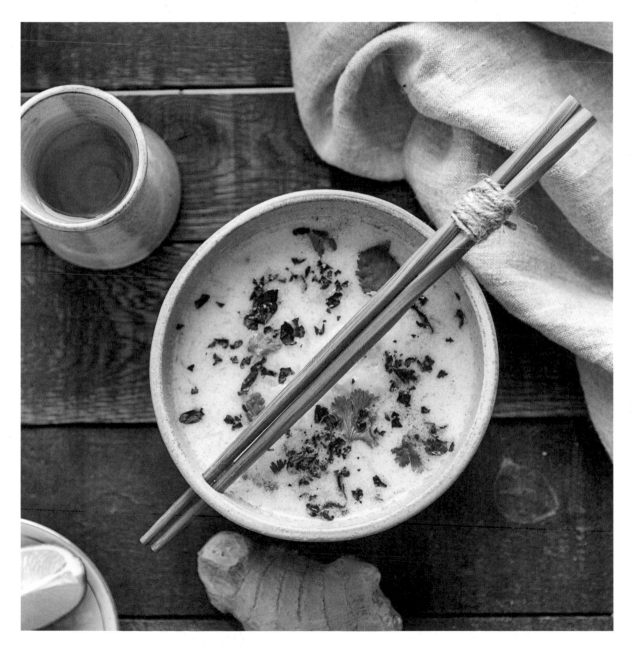

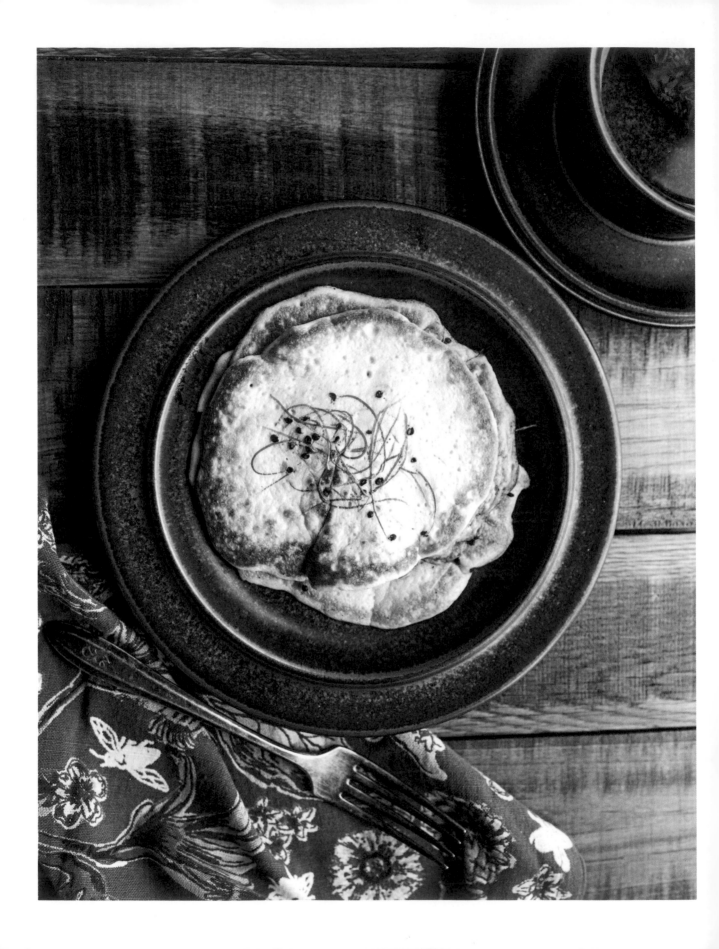

COCONUT-SCALLION PANCAKES

🕐 15 MINUTES   2 🍽   VEGETARIAN 🌿

This recipe for coconut-scallion pancakes, a variation of the subtly sweeter recipe on page 167, is satisfyingly savory with the addition of scallions. A small banana gives the pancakes just enough sweetness, without having to add other sugars.

INGREDIENTS

1 small banana

4 eggs

2 tablespoons almond flour

2 tablespoons coconut flour, plus additional as needed

⅕ 13.5 ounce can (2.7 ounces) coconut milk (use the coconut cream at the top)

1 tablespoon coconut oil

½ cup sliced scallions

DIRECTIONS

1. Add the **banana** and **eggs** to a blender and blend on low. Slowly add the **almond flour** and **coconut flour**, and then the **coconut milk**. Blend until the mixture is well integrated. If the mixture is too liquid, add 1 more tablespoon of the coconut flour.

2. Add the **coconut oil** to a nonstick skillet over medium heat. Slowly begin to pour the mixture into the hot skillet, 3–4 tablespoons at a time, to make the pancakes. Sprinkle some **scallions** into the mixture as the pancakes firm up. Cook the pancakes until bubbles start to form, about 2 minutes. Flip the pancakes and lightly brown them on the opposite side. Plate the pancakes and enjoy them while they're hot.

SPAGHETTI SQUASH LATKES

🕐 15 MINUTES　　2 🍽　　VEGETARIAN

Traditionally, latkes are made with potato, but spaghetti squash browns up just as nicely in the skillet, and is less carb-heavy. Adding a small jalapeño to the mix brings up the spiciness factor by a notch or two, so I highly recommend adding a dollop of tangy kefir dressing to cool it down.

INGREDIENTS

2½ tablespoons coconut oil, divided

1 small shallot, diced

1 small jalapeño, diced

1 cup cooked spaghetti squash, excess water squeezed out

1 egg

2 tablespoons coconut flour

¼ cup kefir (optional)

DIRECTIONS

1. Add ½ tablespoon of the **coconut oil** to a medium nonstick skillet and sauté the **shallot** and **jalapeño** over low heat for 2 minutes, until they've softened.

2. Combine the **squash**, **egg**, and **coconut flour** in a large bowl.

3. Add the shallot and jalapeño to the squash mixture in the large bowl, and mix it together.

4. Using the same skillet over medium-high heat, add the remaining 2 tablespoons of the coconut oil for frying.

5. Spoon the squash mixture, 3–4 tablespoons at a time, into the skillet to form latkes, and fry each of them for 3–4 minutes or until they're brown and crispy on the bottom. Flip the latkes and cook them on the other side until they're browned.

6. Carefully transfer the latkes to paper towel to soak up any excess oil. Plate the latkes and add a dollop of **kefir** to each one, if you'd like.

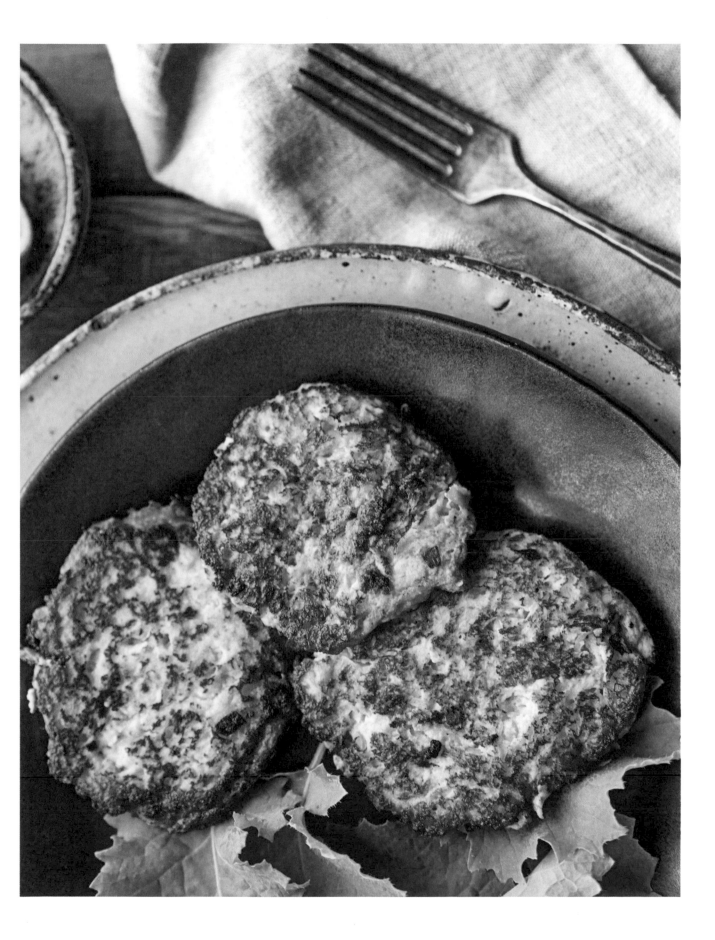

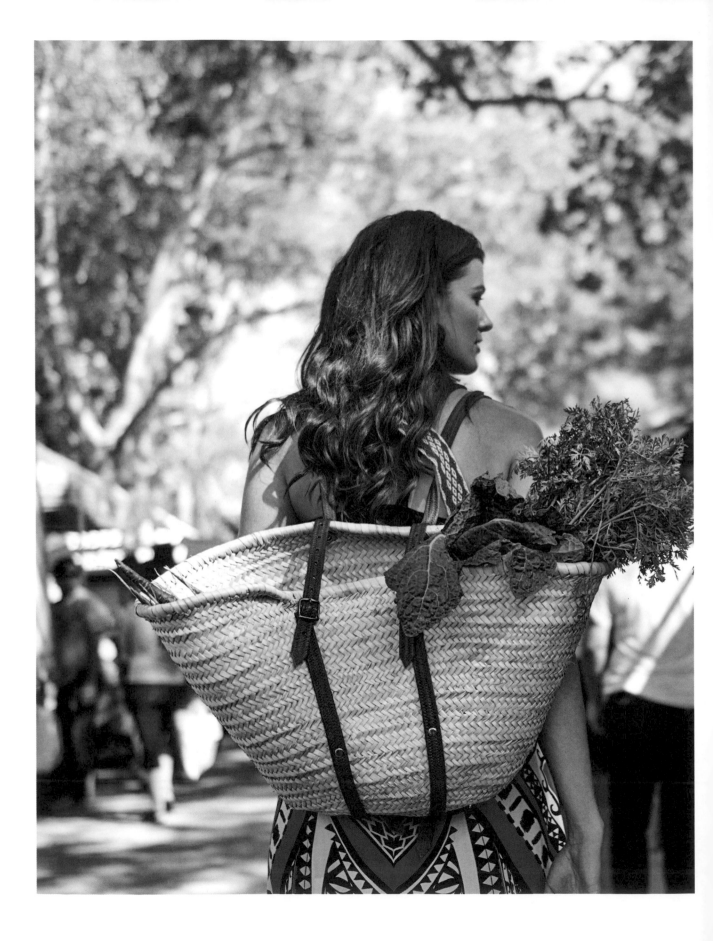

AFTERWORD

Let's All Say Grace

Eating well, as we've learned and probably always intuitively knew, is largely about eating healthy foods that are good for our body, but that's sometimes easier said than done. If it were that simple, then we'd all do it without fail. Instead, we are influenced by all sorts of factors. Some of these are out of our control, like what our parents and grandparents ate well before we were born. And others are seemingly out of our control, like the nearest "good" market or grocery store being 30 miles away (which was the case with one person I spoke with while writing this book), passing by that burger-and-soda billboard on your way to the market, or, once you get to the market, trying to avoid the candy displays at the checkout. Believe me, I tried that—it's hard!

You're likely here, reading this book, because you acknowledge it can be difficult. But you're also here because you know it's possible to change for the better. We want to be healthy for ourselves, and we want to be healthy for the people around us, and we want the people around us to be healthy, too. Paying attention to why we eat and what we eat is like us peering into a tiny keyhole of how we live our life. Once we put that key in and turn it, we're unlocking an opportunity to observe, ask questions about, and even change our lifestyle. Whether we choose to walk through that door and address that fully and with open eyes is ultimately our decision.

Once we make the choice to explore, that's when the learning starts. Some of us may throw up our hands and say, "But I'm so far away from where I want to be!" Great. Even realizing that is an acknowledgment that you are seeking a shift in your life. Voice it more until you're finally provoked to do something about it. As Seneca so sagely advised, "Every new beginning comes from some other beginning's end." You're onto a new beginning as soon as you start thinking differently.

It might not be perfect at first.

It may take more time than you want.

It will require patience. (Lots of it!)

And you'll likely have fits and starts. I consider it *all* progress in the right direction. And you should, too.

Embrace the challenge with the comfort of knowing that cleansing yourself from sugar, eating well, and ultimately living a healthier life is possible. We can shift our lifestyles to become more balanced, allowing space in our life to eat better, and we know now that our food habits are adaptable. We *can* eliminate super-normal stimuli like free sugars to reprogram our brains and recalibrate our taste buds.

We'll start to discover or rediscover our pleasure in food that truly nurtures and nourishes our body. We will hone our taste buds and learn to detect the subtler flavors and sweetness in roasted sweet potatoes, fresh tomatoes, a cob of summer corn, and carrots pulled fresh from the earth. From there, we can begin to take pleasure in our newfound health. If you can imagine it, you can do it.

Every time I sit down for a meal at the dinner table, I feel so grateful that I've not only learned how to eat well and learned how to cook, but also that I am able to share at least some of my good, healthy meals with friends and family. As a matter of fact, sharing meals is a vital component of this book. I knew that if I could share what I was doing with the people that were closest to me, I'd immediately have a wonderful (and thankful!) support group. They, of course, would then pass it on in kind. Even though you and I are not sitting down to a meal together, you did take the time to share in this book, which is very much a part of me. So, I now consider you a part of my extended family of good eaters and aspiring good eaters, and I hope you consider me part of your family as well!

APPENDIX A: THE WHEEL OF LIFE® EXERCISE

Coming to terms with your sugar tooth involves more than knowing what to eat. If it were that simple, then you probably wouldn't make the decision to grab some of those honey-roasted peanuts and a soda when you're hitting a midday slump at work or school. Even when I was working in an office for the better part of a year, I found myself snacking—and sometimes not on the healthiest snacks. Why is that? It wasn't because I really needed or even wanted a snack, but because I was bored of sitting, mindlessly typing emails at my desk. I needed a break, and going to the kitchen was a good enough excuse to get up. These are the types of observations that will be important for you to make in your own life. What are the habits, routines, and triggers that are keeping you from being truly healthy? It becomes an exercise in mindfulness. And mindfulness, like any exercise, takes practice.

The Wheel of Life is an exercise traditionally used by life coaches and a powerful visualization tool that can help bring your life back in balance. I first learned about this useful exercise from a nutritionist friend of mine. If you find that you're snacking and eating depending on how you feel after a tough day at work or whenever your ex's photos pop up in your Facebook feed when you're feeling particularly low, some unhealthy eating habits can kick in. The Wheel of Life exercise can help. Opening up better forms of communication with your colleagues or temporarily blocking your ex from your feed will offer some respite, but the exercise can also help you dig deeper and become more positively proactive in your life, like finally gathering your courage to make a career transition or practicing forgiveness with your ex. Any of those changes will likely transport you to new heights and result in a more balanced life, too.

The wheel represents your whole life and typically contains eight sections, although it can often include more. Each section measures your level of satisfaction in the areas you list, ranging from 0 (not satisfied at all) to 10 (extremely satisfied). It's not a projection of the past or the future. It is simply a snapshot of the present moment. You'll find that your Wheel of Life will vary, sometimes month by month or even day by day. As a matter of fact, at the time of writing this section, I did a Wheel of Life exercise for myself, and my wheel seemed relatively balanced, although it could definitely use improvement in some areas. However, if you had asked me to do the wheel 11 months earlier, I would have had a very different wheel—and it would have been a bumpier trip, as revealed by my eating patterns at the time!

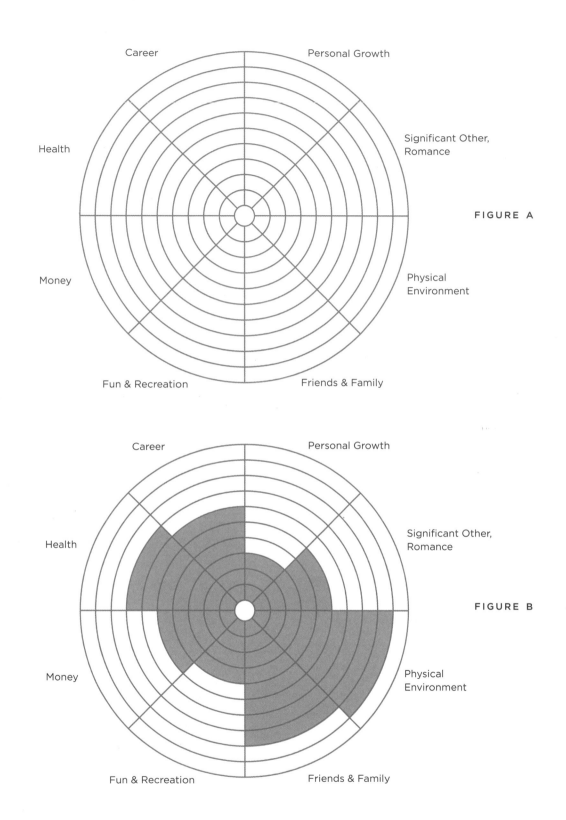

FIGURE A

FIGURE B

The Wheel of Life is a powerful visualization tool to help us determine where we are currently as it relates to living a balanced life. Fill out Figure A to see your own individual wheel.

Figure B is an example of an imaginary Wheel of Life to give you an idea how to fill one out. Where do you think this person can use the most help balancing out his/her life?

How does your Wheel of Life look? Where can you use the most improvement when it comes to balance? How can you become more mindful about that situation, and what are the activities that you need to work on to improve? You may not have those questions at the present moment, and this book doesn't necessarily give you those answers, but it's a simple exercise of mindfulness that can be repeated regularly to help us refocus on ourselves and come to terms with where we may falter, even when we have all the desire to *want* to eat better.

APPENDIX B: HOW TO USE THE YALE FOOD ADDICTION SCALE

The initial score is a symptom count that reflects the number of addiction-like symptoms you have. You may have no symptoms or as many as eleven. I found it particularly useful to have this information because I could then tailor my eating habits to combat those particular symptoms. The YFAS also has a diagnosis score, which indicates whether you qualify for a food addiction and whether it's mild, moderate, or severe.

Now let's get down to business and see where you fall on the YFAS scale!

When you are asked about "certain foods," please think of any foods or beverages that you have had difficulty with in the past 12 months, like sweets such as ice cream, pastries, cookies, cakes, and candies; starches such as bread, pasta, and rice; salty snacks such as chips, pretzels, and crackers; sugary drinks such as sodas, juices, smoothies, lemonade, and sports drinks; and even fatty foods such as pizza and French fries.

IN THE PAST 12 MONTHS:	Never	Less than monthly	Once a month	2–3 times a month	Once a week	2–3 times a week	4–6 times a week	Every Day
1. When I started to eat certain foods, I ate much more than planned. (A)	0	1	2	3	4	5	6	7
2. I continued to eat certain foods even though I was no longer hungry. (A)	0	1	2	3	4	5	6	7

IN THE PAST 12 MONTHS:	Never	Less than monthly	Once a month	2–3 times a month	Once a week	2–3 times a week	4–6 times a week	Every Day
3. I ate to the point where I felt physically ill. (A)	0	1	2	3	4	5	6	7
4. I worried a lot about cutting down on certain types of food, but I ate them anyway. (B)	0	1	2	3	4	5	6	7
5. I spent a lot of time feeling sluggish or tired from overeating. (C)	0	1	2	3	4	5	6	7
6. I spent a lot of time eating certain foods throughout the day. (C)	0	1	2	3	4	5	6	7
7. When certain foods were not available, I went out of my way to get them. For example, I went to the store to get certain foods even though I had other things to eat at home. (C)	0	1	2	3	4	5	6	7
8. I ate certain foods so often or in such large amounts that I stopped doing other important things. These things may have been working or spending time with family or friends. (D)	0	1	2	3	4	5	6	7

IN THE PAST 12 MONTHS:	Never	Less than monthly	Once a month	2-3 times a month	Once a week	2-3 times a week	4-6 times a week	Every Day
9. I had problems with my family or friends because of how much I overate. (H)	0	1	2	3	4	5	6	7
10. I avoided work, school, or social activities because I was afraid I would overeat there. (D)	0	1	2	3	4	5	6	7
11. When I cut down on or stopped eating certain foods, I felt irritable, nervous, or sad. (G)	0	1	2	3	4	5	6	7
12. If I had physical symptoms because I hadn't eaten certain foods, I would eat those foods to feel better. (G)	0	1	2	3	4	5	6	7
13. If I had emotional problems because I hadn't eaten certain foods, I would eat those foods to feel better. (G)	0	1	2	3	4	5	6	7
14. When I cut down on or stopped eating certain foods, I had physical symptoms. For example, I had headaches or fatigue. (G)	0	1	2	3	4	5	6	7

IN THE PAST 12 MONTHS:	Never	Less than monthly	Once a month	2-3 times a month	Once a week	2-3 times a week	4-6 times a week	Every Day
15. When I cut down on or stopped eating certain foods, I had strong cravings for them. (G)	0	1	2	3	4	5	6	7
16. My eating behavior caused me a lot of distress. (L)	0	1	2	3	4	5	6	7
17. I had significant problems in my life because of food and eating. These may have been problems with my daily routine, work, school, friends, family, or health. (L)	0	1	2	3	4	5	6	7
18. I felt so bad about overeating that I didn't do other important things. These things may have been working or spending time with family or friends. (D)	0	1	2	3	4	5	6	7
19. My overeating got in the way of me taking care of my family or doing household chores. (I)	0	1	2	3	4	5	6	7

IN THE PAST 12 MONTHS:	Never	Less than monthly	Once a month	2–3 times a month	Once a week	2–3 times a week	4–6 times a week	Every Day
20. I avoided work, school, or social functions because I could not eat certain foods there. (D)	0	1	2	3	4	5	6	7
21. I avoided social situations because people wouldn't approve of how much I ate. (H)	0	1	2	3	4	5	6	7
22. I kept eating in the same way even though my eating caused emotional problems. (E)	0	1	2	3	4	5	6	7
23. I kept eating the same way even though my eating caused physical problems. (E)	0	1	2	3	4	5	6	7
24. Eating the same amount of food did not give me as much enjoyment as it used to. (F)	0	1	2	3	4	5	6	7
25. I really wanted to cut down on or stop eating certain kinds of foods, but I just couldn't. (B)	0	1	2	3	4	5	6	7

IN THE PAST 12 MONTHS:	Never	Less than monthly	Once a month	2-3 times a month	Once a week	2-3 times a week	4-6 times a week	Every Day
26. I needed to eat more and more to get the feelings I wanted from eating. This included reducing negative emotions like sadness or increasing pleasure. (F)	0	1	2	3	4	5	6	7
27. I didn't do well at work or school because I was eating too much. (I)	0	1	2	3	4	5	6	7
28. I kept eating certain foods even though I knew it was physically dangerous. For example, I kept eating sweets even though I had diabetes, or I kept eating fatty foods despite having heart disease. (J)	0	1	2	3	4	5	6	7
29. I had such strong urges to eat certain foods that I couldn't think of anything else. (K)	0	1	2	3	4	5	6	7
30. I had such intense cravings for certain foods that I felt like I had to eat them right away. (K)	0	1	2	3	4	5	6	7

IN THE PAST 12 MONTHS:	Never	Less than monthly	Once a month	2–3 times a month	Once a week	2–3 times a week	4–6 times a week	Every Day
31. I tried to cut down on or not eat certain kinds of food, but I wasn't successful. (B)	0	1	2	3	4	5	6	7
32. I tried and failed to cut down on or stop eating certain foods. (B)	0	1	2	3	4	5	6	7
33. I was so distracted by eating that I could have been hurt (e.g., when driving a car, crossing the street, operating machinery. (J)	0	1	2	3	4	5	6	7
34. I was so distracted by thinking about food that I could have been hurt (e.g., when driving a car, crossing the street, operating machinery). (J)	0	1	2	3	4	5	6	7
35. My friends or family were worried about how much I overate. (H)	0	1	2	3	4	5	6	7

Here's how the scoring works.

Questions are grouped by **symptom criteria.**

> A. Substance taken in larger amount and for longer period than intended: questions 1, 2, 3
>
> B. Persistent desire or repeated unsuccessful attempts to quit: questions 4, 25, 31, 32
>
> C. Much time/activity to obtain, use, recover: questions 5, 6, 7
>
> D. Important social, occupational, or recreational activities given up or reduced: questions 8, 10, 18, 20
>
> E. Use continues despite knowledge of adverse consequences (e.g., emotional problems, physical problems): questions 22, 23
>
> F. Tolerance (marked increase in amount consumed; marked decrease in effect): questions 24, 2
>
> G. Characteristic withdrawal symptoms; substance taken to relieve withdrawal: questions 11, 12, 13, 14,
>
> H. Continued use despite social or interpersonal problems: questions 9, 21, 35
>
> I. Failure to fulfill major role obligation (e.g., work, school, home): questions 19, 27
>
> J. Use in physically hazardous situations: questions 28, 33, 34
>
> K. Craving, or a strong desire or urge to use: questions 29, 30
>
> L. Use causes clinically significant impairment or distress: questions 16, 17

Each question has a different threshold whereby 0 = threshold not met and 1 = threshold is met. The thresholds vary by each question and are grouped in the following ways:

1. Once a month: 9, 10, 19, 27, 33, 35
2. Two to three times a month: 8, 18, 20, 21, 34
3. Once a week: 3, 11, 13, 14, 22, 28, 29
4. Two to three times a week: 5, 12, 16, 17, 23, 24, 26, 30, 31, 32
5. Four to six times a week: 1, 2, 4, 6, 7, 15, 25

After computing the threshold for each question, add up the scores for the questions under each criterion (e.g., tolerance, withdrawal, clinical significance, etc.). If the score for the symptom criterion is less than 1, then the criterion has been met and is scored as 1. If the score is 0, then the symptom criterion has not been met and is scored as 0.

EXAMPLE:

> Tolerance: (question 24 = 1) + (question 26 = 0) = 1, criterion met
>
> Craving: (question 29 = 0) + (question 30 = 0), criterion not met

Now we are going to see how many symptoms we have. Add up all of the scores for each of the eleven criteria. Do not add clinical significance to the score. This score should range from zero symptoms to eleven symptoms.

Finally, in order to "diagnose" whether you have an addiction, both the symptom count score and the clinical significance criteria are used.

No food addiction = 1 or fewer symptoms

No food addiction = Does not meet criteria for clinical significance

Mild food addiction = 2 or 3 symptoms and clinical significance

Moderate food addiction = 4 or 5 symptoms and clinical significance

Severe food addiction = 6 or more symptoms and clinical significance

Though the YFAS is an involved scoring process, it gives you a more accurate sense as to which symptoms you exhibit and how they are affecting your life, and it allows you to improve or resolve the issues through a more informed approach.

APPENDIX C. SUGAR'S MANY NAMES

Part of becoming savvy about sugar is learning how to read nutrition labels. What can make this challenging, however, is the fact that sugar, sugar alcohols, and artificial sweeteners hide behind many different names. Here's a comprehensive, though not exhaustive list of some of them:

Acesulfame	Dextrose	Maple syrup
Acesulfame potassium	Diastatic malt	Molasses
Agave nectar	Diatase	Monk fruit
Agave syrup	Erythritol	Muscovado sugar
Aspartame	Ethyl maltol	Neotame
Barbados sugar	Evaporated cane juice	Organic raw sugar
Barley malt	Florida crystals	Panocha
Beet sugar	Fructose	Polydextrose
Blackstrap molasses	Fruit juice	Raw sugar
Brown rice syrup	Fruit juice concentrate	Refiner's syrup
Brown sugar	Galactose	Rice syrup
Buttered syrup	Glucose	Saccharin
Cane juice	Glucose solids	Sorbitol
Cane juice crystals	Golden sugar	Sorghum syrup
Cane sugar	Golden syrup	Stevia
Caramel	Grape juice	Sucanat
Carob syrup	Grape sugar	Sucralose
Castor sugar	High-fructose corn syrup	Sucrose
Confectioner's sugar	Honey	Sugar
Corn sweetener	Icing sugar	Treacle
Corn syrup	Invert sugar	Turbinado sugar
Corn syrup solids	Lactose	Yellow sugar
Crystalline fructose	Malt syrup	Xylitol
Date sugar	Maltodextrin	Zerose
Demerara sugar	Maltose	
Dextran	Manitol	

APPENDIX D. SHOPPING LIST

Here is a shopping list of preferred ingredients. The items in red symbolize fruits and vegetables that are particularly high in natural sugars or starch, which means you should try not to consume more than ½ cup or 1 serving of them per day. If you are vegan or vegetarian, you can substitute meats with tempeh, tofu, or beans; cheeses with nut butters; yogurts with non-dairy coconut yogurt; and any creams with avocado or coconut milk.

VEGETABLES
Artichokes
Arugula (rocket)
Asparagus*
Bamboo shoots
Beet greens
Beets*
Bell peppers
Bok choy
Broccoli
Broccolini
Broccoli rabe
Brussels sprouts
Cabbage
Carrot
Cauliflower
Celeriac
Celery
Chard
Chicory root*
Collards
Corn
Daikon
Dandelion greens*
Endive
Fennel
Garlic*
Ginger
Hot pepper
Jerusalem artichoke*
Jicama*
Kale

Kohlrabi
Leeks*
Lettuce
Microgreens
Mustard greens
Nori/seaweed
Onion, red*
Onion, scallion
Onion, shallot*
Onion, white*
Onion, yellow*
Parsley root
Parsnips
Potato
Potato, sweet
Purslane
Radicchio
Radish
Rhubarb
Romaine lettuce
Rutabaga
Spinach
Sprouts
Taro
Turnip
Turnip greens
Water chestnuts
Watercress
Yams

MUSHROOMS
All edible mushrooms

HERBS
All herbs

SPICES
All spices

FRUITS**
Apricot
Avocado
Banana
Blackberry
Blueberry
Chiles
Coconut
Cucumber
Eggplant (aubergine)
Grapefruit
Lemon
Lime
Melons
Nectarine
Okra
Olives*
Orange
Peach
Peppers
Plum
Pumpkin
Squash, acorn
Squash, buttercup
Squash, butternut
Squash, delicata

Squash, kombocha

Squash, spaghetti

Raspberry

Strawberry

String beans

Tangerine

Tomatillo

Tomatoes

Watermelon

Zucchini, green

Zucchini, yellow

NUTS, SEEDS & NUT BUTTERS

Almonds

Almond butter

Cashews

Chestnuts

Chia seeds

Flax seeds

Hazelnuts

Hemp seeds

Macadamia nuts

Pecans

Pine nuts

Pistachios*

Pumpkin seeds

Sesame seeds

Sunflower seeds

Tahini

Walnuts

FATS AND OILS

Animal fat (grass-fed, organic)

Avocado oil

Coconut butter

Coconut oil

Extra virgin olive oil

Flaxseed oil, unrefined and expeller pressed

Ghee

Macadamia butter

Sesame oil

MEATS AND ANIMAL-BASED PROTEIN

Eggs (pastured, organic)

Ham

Poultry (pastured, organic)

Beef, lamb, venison (100% grass-fed, organic)

Pork

Rabbit (pastured, organic)

Offal

Shellfish

Seafood (wild-caught, sustainably harvested)

Venison and game animals

GRAINS AND LEGUMES

Barley, pearl

Black beans

Black-eyed peas

Chickpeas

Edamame

Fava beans

Kidney beans

Lentils

Lima beans

Mung beans

Navy beans

Peas, snow

Peas, sugar snap

Pinto beans

Quinoa

Red beans

Rice, brown

Split peas

White beans

BREAD

Sourdough, fresh

Rye

DAIRY

Cheese: hard cheeses, feta, raw cheese (keep to a small matchbox portion/day)

Non-dairy, coconut milk yogurt

Non-dairy, coconut milk

Non-dairy, nut milk

Cottage cheese, plain

Crème fraîche

Goat's milk kefir, plain

Greek yogurt, plain

Mozzarella, fresh (keep to 6 ounces)

Sour cream

BAKING INGREDIENTS

Almond flour

Baking powder

Baking soda

Carob powder

Coconut flour

Garbanzo flour

Vanilla extract

Yeast

SPECIALTY PRODUCTS

Dark chocolate (70% minimum cocoa content)

Sweet white miso or similar miso

Tamari Sauce

* Foods beneficial for good gut health.

** Some items listed as "fruit" are traditionally eaten as vegetables, but they are technically fruit. The easiest way to tell the difference is that fruits have seeds.

APPENDIX E. FRUITS AND FRUIT SUGARS

The table below lists the total number of sugars and the total amount of fructose in a single serving of fruit, from the lowest fructose level to the highest. Please note that this is a comprehensive but by no means exhaustive list. Additionally, fruit sugars vary from fruit to fruit, so consider the totals as estimates. Finally, certain studies, though limited, show that eating whole fruits can have positive effects on your body, regardless of how many servings you eat, so if you find yourself eating more fresh fruits in the summer months, that's okay!

	Total Sugars (mg)	Fructose (mg)
Avocado	0.9	0.2
Lime	0.4	0.2
Apricots	9.3	0.7
Lemon	2.5	0.8
Grapefruit, pink	6.2	1.2
Grapefruit, white	6.2	1.2
Peach	8.7	1.3
Jackfruit	8.4	1.4
Tomato	2.8	1.4
Cantaloupe	8.7	1.8
Plum	7.5	1.8
Guava, strawberry	6	1.9
Guava	6	1.9
Pineapple	11.9	2.1
Orange	9.2	2.5
Strawberries	5.8	2.5
Banana	15.6	2.7
Papaya	5.9	2.7
Figs	6.9	2.8
Mango	14.8	2.9
Purple passion fruit or granadilla	11.2	3.1
Raspberries	9.5	3.2
Starfruit	7.1	3.2
Cherries, sour	8.1	3.3
Watermelon	9	3.3

Blueberries	7.3	3.6
Mamey apple	6.5	3.7
Blackberries	8.1	4.1
Kiwi fruit	10.5	4.3
Maple sugar	85.2	4.3
Pomegranate	10.1	4.7
Cherries, sweet	14.6	6.2
Pear, Bosc	10.5	6.4
Apples	13.3	7.6
Grapes	18.1	7.6
Dried apricots	38.9	12.2
Dried prunes	44	14.8
Dried peaches	44.6	15.6
Dates	64.2	22.3
Dried figs	62.3	24.4
Raisins, regular	65	33.8
Raisins, golden	70.6	37.1
Zante currants	70.6	37.1

BIBLIOGRAPHY

Advertising Age. 2014. Data Center, Marketer Family Trees 2013 Update, Kellogg Co. http://adage.com/datacenter/marketertrees2013update/#62. Accessed July 31, 2016.

Avena, N. M., et al. 2005. Sugar-Dependent Rats Show Enhanced Responding for Sugar after Abstinence: Evidence of a Sugar Deprivation Effect. *Physiology and Behavior* 84(3):359–362. http://www.sciencedirect.com/science/article/pii/S0031938405000065 Accessed July 31, 2016.

Avena, N. M., et al. 2011. Animal Models of Sugar and Fat Bingeing: Relationship to Food Addiction and Increased Body Weight. *Psychiatric Disorders* 829: 351–365 http://link.springer.com/protocol/10.1007/978-1-61779-458-2_23. Accessed July 31, 2016.

Babey, S., et al. 2016. Prediabetes in California: Nearly Half of California Adults on Path to Diabetes [report]. UCLA Center for Health Policy Research. http://healthpolicy.ucla.edu/publications/Documents/PDF/2016/prediabetes-brief-mar2016.pdf. Accessed August 2, 2016.

Bailin, et al. 2014. Sugar-coating Science: How the Food Industry Misleads Consumers on Sugar [report]. Cambridge, MA: Center for Science and Democracy, Union of Concerned Scientists. Pp. 2–5. http://www.ucsusa.org/sites/default/files/legacy/assets/documents/center-for-science-and-democracy/sugar-coating-science.pdf. Accessed July 31, 2016.

Bartolotto, C. 2015. Does Consuming Sugar and Artificial Sweeteners Change Taste Preferences? *Permanente Journal* 19(3):81–84. http://www.thepermanentejournal.org/issues/50-the-permanente-journal/commentary/5893-sugar.html. Accessed August 2, 2016.

Bayol, S. A., et al. 2007. A Maternal 'Junk Food' Diet in Pregnancy and Lactation Promotes an Exacerbated Taste for 'Junk Food' and a Greater Propensity for Obesity in Rat Offspring. *British Journal of Nutrition* 98(4): 843–851. http://journals.cambridge.org/action/displayAbstract?fromPage=online&aid=1343304&fileId=S0007114507812037. Accessed July 31, 2016.

Beauchamp, G. K., and J. A. Mennelia. 2009. Early Flavor Learning and Its Impact on Later Feeding Behavior. *Journal of Pediatric Gastroenterology and Nutrition*. 48:S25–S30. http://journals.lww.com/jpgn/Abstract/2009/03001/Early_Flavor_Learning_and_Its_Impact_on_Later.5.aspx. Accessed July 17, 2016.

Belluz, Julia. 2016. The FDA Just Made the Most Significant Changes to the Nutrition Label in Years. Vox, May 20, 2016. http://www.vox.com/2016/5/20/11719796/new-nutrition-label-added-sugar. Accessed July 31, 2016.

Boyland, E. J., et al., 2016. Advertising as a Cue to Consume: A Systematic Review and Meta-Analysis of the Effects of Acute Exposure to Unhealthy Food and Nonalcoholic Beverage Advertising on Intake in Children and Adults. *American Journal of Clinical Nutrition*, January 20. http://ajcn.nutrition.org/content/early/2016/01/20/ajcn.115.120022.short. Accessed July 31, 2016.

Carr, Abigail. 2013. *Three Squares: The Invention of the American Meal*. New York: Basic Books.

Credit Suisse. 2013. Sugar Consumption at a Crossroads [report]. P. 38. https://publications.credit-suisse.com/tasks/render/file/index.cfm?fileid=780BF4A8-B3D1-13A0-D2514E21EFFB0479. Accessed July 31, 2016.

Cuda-Kroen, Gretchen. 2011. Baby's Palate and Food Memories Shaped before Birth. NPR Morning Edition, August 8. http://www.npr.org/2011/08/08/139033757/babys-palate-and-food-memories-shaped-before-birth. Accessed July 31, 2016.

Fleming, A. 2014. How a Child's Food Preferences Begin in the Womb. *Guardian*, April 8. https://www.theguardian.com/lifeandstyle/wordofmouth/2014/apr/08/child-food-preferences-womb-pregnancy-foetus-taste-flavours. Accessed July 31, 2016.

Fokazi, S. 2012. Sugar Addiction Programme Launched. IOL, October 18. http://www.iol.co.za/lifestyle/sugar-addiction-programme-launched-1405933. Accessed July 31, 2016.

Food and Addiction Science and Treatment Lab. Yale Food Addiction Scale. http://fastlab.psych.lsa.umich.edu/yale-food-addiction-scale/. Accessed July 31, 2016

Gallagher, J. 2016. Deadly Diabetes in an 'Unrelenting March.' BBC News, April 6. http://www.bbc.com/news/health-35959554. Accessed July 31, 2016.

Garvan Institute of Medical Research. 2016 Jul 18. Grandpa's Obesity Affects the Health of His Grandchildren: Mouse Study. Science Daily, July 18. https://www.sciencedaily.com/releases/2016/07/160718110933.htm. Accessed July 31, 2016.

Gearhardt, A. N., et al., 2014. Relation of Obesity to Neural Activation in Response to Food Commercials. *Social Cognitive and Affective Neuroscience*, July 9(7):932–938. http://www.ncbi.nlm.nih.gov/pubmed/23576811. Accessed July 31, 2016.

Haber, G. B., et al. 1977. Depletion and Disruption of Dietary Fibre: Effects of Satiety, Plasma-Glucose, and Serum-Insulin. *Lancet* 310(8040): 679–689. http://www.sciencedirect.com/science/article/pii/S0140673677904949. Accessed July 31, 2016.

Hadhazy, A. 2010. Think Twice: How the Gut's "Second Brain" Influences Mood and Well-Being. *Scientific American*, February 12. http://www.scientificamerican.com/article/gut-second-brain/. Accessed July 31, 2016.

Hanks, A., et al. 2016. Marketing Vegetables in Elementary School Cafeterias to Increase Uptake. *Pediatrics*. 138(2) 1–9. http://pediatrics.aappublications.org/content/pediatrics/early/2016/07/01/peds.2015-1720.full.pdf. Accessed August 11, 2016.

Ifland, J. R., et al. 2009. Refined Food Addiction: A Classic Substance Use Disorder. *Medical Hypotheses* 72(5):518–526. http://www.sciencedirect.com/science/article/pii/S0306987708006427. Accessed July 31, 2016.

Jabr, Ferris. 2013. How the Brain Gets Addicted to Gambling. *Scientific American*, November 1. http://www.scientificamerican.com/article/how-the-brain-gets-addicted-to-gambling/. Accessed August 12, 2016.

Kraak, V. I., and M. Story. 2014. Influence of Food Companies' Brand Mascots and Entertainment Companies' Cartoon Media Characters on Children's Diet and Health: A Systematic Review and Research Needs. *Obesity Reviews*, December 17. http://onlinelibrary.wiley.com/doi/10.1111/obr.12237/full.

Lustig, Robert H., et al. 2015. Isocaloric Fructose Restriction and Metabolic Improvement in Children with Obesity and Metabolic Syndrome. *Obesity*, October 26. http://onlinelibrary.wiley.com/doi/10.1002/oby.21371/abstract. Accessed July 31, 2016.

McClear, S. 2014. Experts Say Juice Cleanses Are Unnecessary, Expensive, and Often Packed with Sugar. *New York Daily News*, July 11. http://www.nydailynews.com/life-style/juice-fasts-cleansed-sense-article-1.1862531.

Meule, A., and A. N. Gearhardt. 2014. Five Years of the Yale Food Addiction Scale: Taking Stock and Moving Forward. *Current Addiction Reports*, May 10. http://fastlab.psych.lsa.umich.edu/wp-content/uploads/2014/06/MeuleGearhardt_FiveYearsoftheYaleFoodAddictionScale-TakingStockMovingForward_2014.pdf Accessed July 31, 2016.

Moynihan, P., and P. E. Petersen. 2004. Diet, Nutrition, and the Prevention of Dental Diseases. *Public Health Nutrition* 7(1A): 201–226. http://www.who.int/nutrition/publications/public_health_nut7.pdf. Accessed August 4, 2016.

Munro, D. 2013. Sugar Linked to $1 Trillion in U.S. Healthcare Spending. Forbes.com, October 27. http://www.forbes.com/sites/danmunro/2013/10/27/sugar-linked-to-1-trillion-in-u-s-healthcare-spending/#70f875d82058. Accessed July 31, 2016.

National Sustainable Agriculture Coalition. 2016. Release: USDA Revokes Grass Fed Label Standard [press release]. January 12. http://sustainableagriculture.net/blog/release-usda-revokes-grass-fed-label-standard/.

New America. Federal Education Budget Overview. November 12, 2015. http://atlas.newamerica.org/education-federal-budget. Accessed July 31, 2016.

Owen, N., et al. 2010. Sedentary Behavior: Emerging Evidence for a New Health Risk. *Mayo Clinical Proceedings*. 85(12): 1138–1141. http://www.ncbi.nlm.nih.gov/pmc/articles/PMC2996155/. Accessed July 31, 2016.

Popkin, B. M. 2015. Sugar Consumption in the Food and Beverage Supply across the Globe. In *Dietary Sugars and Health*, edited by M. I. Goran et al. Boca Raton, FL: CRC Press. Pp. 127–128.

Saben, J. L. 2016. Maternal Metabolic Syndrome Programs Mitochondrial Dysfunction via Germline Changes across Three Generations [report]. http://www.cell.com/cell-reports/pdf/S2211-1247(16)30663-5.pdf. Accessed August 2, 2016.

U.S. Department of Agriculture, Economic Research Service. 2015. USDA Sugar Supply: Tables 51-53: US Consumption of Caloric Sweeteners. http://www.ers.usda.gov/data-products/sugar-and-sweeteners-yearbook-tables.aspx. Accessed October 5, 2016.

U.S. Department of Agriculture and U.S. Department of Health and Human Services. 2010. Dietary Guidelines for Americans. https://health.gov/dietaryguidelines/dga2010/DietaryGuidelines2010.pdf. Accessed July 31, 2016.

Vartanian, L. R., et al. 2016. Clutter, Chaos, and Overconsumption: The Role of Mind-Set in Stressful and Chaotic Food Environments. *Environment and Behavior*, February. http://eab.sagepub.com/content/early/2016/01/28/0013916516628178.abstract. Accessed on July 31, 2016.

Wansink, B., et al. 2015. Slim by Design: Kitchen Counter Correlates of Obesity. *Health Education and Behavior*. http://heb.sagepub.com/content/early/2015/10/15/1090198115610571.full. Accessed August 12, 2016.

Wharton, C. M. et al. 2014. Dietary Self-Monitoring, but Not Dietary Quality, Improves with Use of Smartphone App Technology in an 8-Week Weight Loss Trial. *Journal of Nutrition Education and Behavior* 46(5): 440–444. http://www.sciencedirect.com/science/article/pii/S1499404614004692. Accessed July 31, 2016.

World Health Organization. 2015. Guideline: Sugars Intake for Adults and Children. http://www.who.int/nutrition/publications/guidelines/sugars_intake/en/. Accessed August 2, 2016.

RESOURCES

INSTITUTIONS AND ORGANIZATIONS

Center for Science in the Public Interest (CSPI)
https://cspinet.org

Eat Tank
http://www.eattank.org

Environmental Working Group
http://www.ewg.org

Food and Addiction Science and Treatment Lab
http://fastlab.psych.lsa.umich.edu

Food Policy Action
http://foodpolicyaction.org

Food Tank
http://foodtank.com

Institute for Responsible Nutrition
http://www.responsiblefoods.org

Jamie Oliver Food Foundation
http://www.jamiesfoodrevolution.org

National Institutes of Health
https://www.nih.gov

The Noakes Foundation
http://www.thenoakesfoundation.org

Nutrition Science Initiative
http://nusi.org

Sugar Science
http://www.sugarscience.org

Uconn Rudd Center for Food Policy and Obesity
http://www.uconnruddcenter.org

United States Healthful Food Council
http://ushfc.org

DIABETES INFORMATION
DiaTribe
http://diatribe.org/type-2-diabetes

American Diabetes Association
http://www.diabetes.org

SUGAR ADDICTION TREATMENT
Elements Behavioral Health
https://www.elementsbehavioralhealth.com

Healthy Eating and Lifestyle Program
http://www.helpdiet.co.za

Malibu Vista
https://www.malibuvista.com

Renascent
http://renascent.ca

BOOKS

Carroll, Abigail. *Three Squares: The Invention of the American Meal.* New York: Basic Books, 2013.

Duhigg, Charles. *The Power of Habit: Why We Do What We Do in Life and Business.* New York: Random House, 2012.

Goran, Michael I., Luc Tappy, and Kim-Anne Lê, eds. *Dietary Sugars and Health.* Boca Raton, FL: CRC Press, 2015.

Hyman, Mark. *The Blood Sugar Solution: The UltraHealthy Program for Losing Weight, Preventing Disease, and Feeling Great Now!* New York: Little, Brown and Co., 2012.

Lustig, Robert H. *Fat Chance: Beating the Odds against Sugar, Processed Food, Obesity, and Disease.* New York: Plume, 2013.

Moss, Michael. *Salt, Sugar, Fat: How the Food Giants Hooked Us.* New York: Random House, 2013.

Nestle, Marion. *Food Politics: How the Food Industry Influences Nutrition and Health*, rev. ed. California Studies in Food and Culture. Berkeley: University of California Press, 2013.

Nestle, Marion. *Soda Politics: Taking on Big Soda (and Winning).* New York: Oxford University Press, 2015.

Pollan, Michael, and Maira Kalman. *Food Rules: An Eater's Manual*, rev. ed. New York: Penguin, 2011.

Wilson, Bee. *First Bite: How We Learn to Eat.* New York: Basic Books, 2015.

ABOUT SUGARDETOX.ME

This book is a part of SugarDetox.me, the website, which provides additional resources and free and affordable sugar cleanse programs. Visit SugarDetox.me and follow us at your preferred locations on social media.

Facebook: https://www.facebook.com/sugardetoxme

Instagram: instagram.com/srmanitou and instagram.com/sugardetoxme

Twitter: @sroakes

ABOUT THE AUTHOR

Summer Rayne Oakes was reclaiming mine sites, researching sewage sludge, and restoring forestlands when she was struck with the idea that style—and how we live our life—would be a far more effective means to connect people to the natural world. Graduating Cornell University cum laude with degrees in Environmental Science and Entomology, Oakes began to bridge her interest in ecological systems to industries that affect our everyday life—from what we wear to what we eat.

In 2009, while modeling full-time, Oakes cofounded Source4Style (now Le Souk) to connect designers to more sustainable textile suppliers around the globe—from cotton weavers in India to silk spinners in Cambodia. From there she applied her knowledge of global systems and a customer's personal connection to what she buys to a new challenge: Food.

She began to help food start-ups launch their initiatives to build and strengthen more sustainable, regional food systems. While working in the world of good food, Oakes founded SugarDetox.me, a website designed to first help her overcome her sweet tooth, and later to assist people all over the world to cleanse themselves from sugar, and which also inspired this book. The website offers easy-to-follow, affordable cleanses, centered around helping people transition away from sugary, processed foods and to begin embracing whole foods free of added sugars.

Oakes's vision is to help find the extraordinary in people by inspiring and empowering them to live an active, healthy, fulfilling, and sustainable life. Her work has been featured in a range of media outlets worldwide, including: CNN, *The New York Times*, *The Guardian*, *Vogue*, *Vanity Fair*, *INC*, and others. You may see her in Brooklyn cooking sugar-free meals, hanging out at her local community garden, or tending to her own copious indoor jungle. More about her work can be found at www.summerrayne.net and www.sugardetox.me.

ACKNOWLEDGMENTS

In the fast-paced environment of city life—it's not unusual to go out to grab drinks and a meal with friends. It is, however, pretty unusual to stay at home and cook. Though I grew up with meals around the table—my current environment in the city has made cooking for others in my home something of a novelty, something special. As such, I would like to thank **all my friends** who have gathered around my dinner table to share both good conversations and good meals. I know these little gestures have only brought us closer.

I also have to extend the deepest gratitude to my parents—**Bob** and **Diane**—who still, to this day, garden, cook, and stay physically active, as well as my grandparents, **Smittie** and **Lil**. They have instilled the foundation of good eating and good habits in me—and for that, I am forever grateful.

A special thanks is in order to **Tony Gardner**, my literary agent—this book would never have been made possible without his encouragement, guidance and dedication. I can't say thank-you enough! Tony, I admire you for your skill and integrity as an agent, and very much cherish the friendship that this experience has brought. Here's looking to more books to come! To **Scott Feldman**, my agent at Two Twelve Management and Marketing, who introduced me to Tony in the first place—and believed in me from the moment we first met! Thank you for taking a chance on a wild card like me.

A wholehearted thank-you to **Sander van Dijk**—partner, creative counterpart, and friend. You have believed in me and this initiative from the get-go and never wavered in your support. Your creative guidance throughout this process has been indispensable. You have helped me learn how to question everything—in both this project and in life—and have filled many roles throughout this time. Thank you for your creativity, patience, insights, love, friendship, and support. To **Damon Horowitz**, who has been my biggest cheerleader since we met during my first book tour back in May 2009. I really value our relationship—so far beyond what you may ever know. It's all too rare to have people in our lives who not only want to see us be the best, most fulfilled human that we can possibly be—but then go out of their way to fully support that person. You have been that person for me. Thank you for your advice, guidance, and love over these past eight years. I hope to someday be able to return that favor in kind. Of course, I can't leave out my wonderful friend and creative counterpart, **Joey L.** Joey, there was an inevitability to us meeting. You are talent and discipline incarnate. I love and value our time and work together. And I love how we help one another, without hesitation or question; that is true friendship. Thank you for stepping up and stepping in to do some of the photography for the book, and being there as creative guidance along the way.

Ohn Mar Win, your illustrations have really brought vibrancy to the book and the website. Thank you for jumping on board this project. I only hope to meet you in the flesh someday soon! **Bhadresh G.** and **Koen O.**, thank you for giving life to the website; and to **Joey K.** for guiding me through the ropes of the new website design. And to my friends **Zoe Tryon** and **Wade Davis,** who were so gracious to put me in touch with acquaintances that I could run the book by. A hearty thanks to **Leslie Lee** of the Institute for Responsible Nutrition for reading over my book and providing insights into some of the latest sugar science.

To **Team Sterling**: I'm forever grateful that you took on this book and are as excited for it as I am! A special thanks to **Theresa Thompson**, who has been a champion for *SugarDetoxMe* since she first saw it come across her desk. To my editors, **Jennifer Williams,** for being such a gem and incredibly open-minded to my suggestions and changes along the way; and **Marilyn Kretzer**, who stood by the book the whole time to ensure it's the best that it can possibly be whilst navigating through difficult times. Thank you to **Lorie Pagnozzi, Jo Obarowski**, and **Renee Yewdaev** for guiding through the design of the book and **Chris Bain** for organizing all the photography. And of course, all the others who have contributed to the success of this book: **Blanca Oliviery, Sari Lampert, Trudi Bartow, Alexandra Leith, Chris Vaccari,** and anyone else who I have yet to meet or may have left out! Thank you!

A special thanks to **all my friends** who gave feedback on the early book designs; and to all of those who have chosen to put their health first and do the sugar detox programs with me. Your participation and insights are so highly appreciated. Thank you all!

INDEX

Note: Page numbers in *italics* indicate recipes.